GREEN FOODS FOR MEN

GREEN FOODS FOR MEN

MICHAEL DE MEDEIROS
JENNY WESTERKAMP, R.D., L.D.

FAIR WINDS

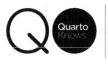

Quarto is the authority on a wide range of topics.

Quarto educates, entertains and enriches the lives of our readers—enthusiasts and lovers of hands-on living.

www.QuartoKnows.com

First published in the USA in 2015 by
Fair Winds Press, an imprint of
Quarto Publishing Group USA Inc.
100 Cummings Center
Suite 406-L
Beverly, MA 01915-6101
QuartoKnows.com
Visit our blogs at QuartoKnows.com

ISBN: 978-1-59233-632-6

Digital edition published in 2015
eISBN: 978-1-62788-176-0

Library of Congress Cataloging-in-Publication Data available

Cover and book design by The Lincoln Avenue Workshop
Photography by Robert Reiff
Food styling by Sandra Cordero
Printed and bound in USA

*The information in this book is for educational purposes only. It is not intended
to replace the advice of a physician or medical practitioner. Please see your
health care provider before beginning any new health program.*

Dedication

For my father. This book has a few of the countless lessons he taught me. And for my brothers. —MDM

For my dad and five brothers, the toughest—and most rewarding— clients I will ever have. —JW

CONTENTS

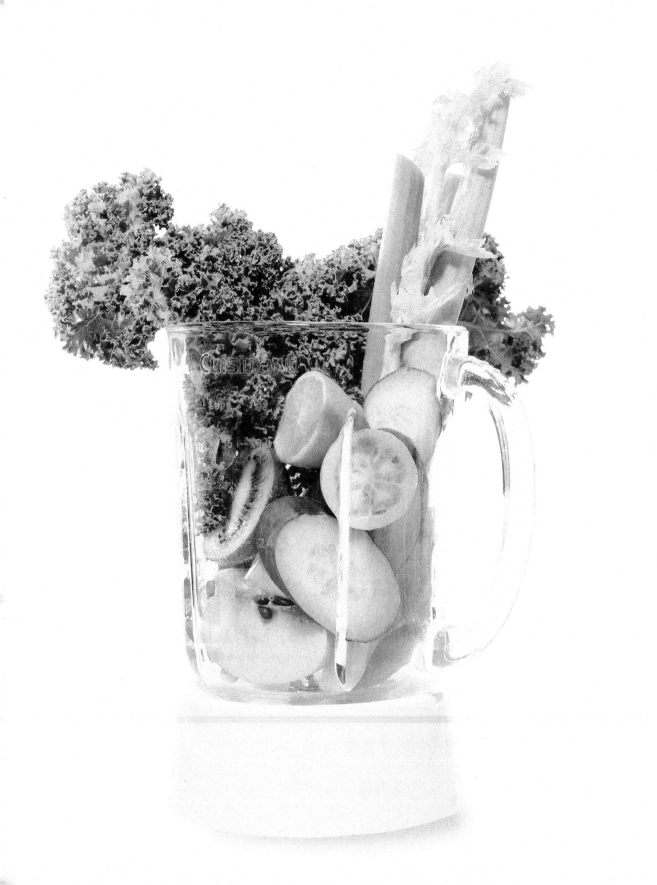

WHY MEN SHOULD EAT GREEN

Few things unite men more than their universal aversion to green foods. From caveman through the ages to today's more refined gent, men have always craved meat, avoided greens, and have been very proud of it. And while man has made millions of advances since his first days on this planet, appreciating the benefits of eating green foods is not one of them. History has recorded it, attitudes explain it, and science proves it.

How eating green foods—vegetables, herbs, plants, fruits, and the like—became unmanly is truly a question that one must consult history to understand. Men through all eras have eaten greens, but the fact that they've done it busting each others' chops about eating vegetables in public only to secretly delight in them in the privacy of their own home. Left alone, those dinner plates may be healthy or unhealthy—that depends on each individual—but they're more often than not partnered with a side of greens.

The truth is men *do* eat their greens—but they're not doing it with any regularity, frequency, or volume. And the reason could simply be their eating habits. In our experience, there are five general types of eaters in the male gender.

THE TANK FILLER: This guy is serious about his nutrition. He eats to fuel his gains in the gym. Food is his catalyst for building muscle. He has at least one protein shake every day. He uses supplements to cover the deficiencies of his diet and counts the grams of each meal. While he does eat some greens, he isn't eating enough—but he's sure he's getting everything he *really* needs to build the body he wants.

THE OVER FILLER: Simply put, this guy eats too much. He's not particularly active, eats without any plan, and steadily gains weight throughout his life. He snacks, he eats big meals late in the evening, and he loves salty, sugary, and fried foods. The only greens he's seeing in his diet are usually drowned in cream or cheese or deep fried. He eats what he wants and doesn't consider himself *too* unhealthy and would probably call you Nancy if you ordered a salad for dinner.

THE UNDER FILLER: Most people think that men aren't capable of obsessing over their diet and assume only women starve themselves. The truth is there are men who are under eating but they aren't doing it for weight loss. Instead, these are men who either ignore hunger or satisfy it with minimal nourishment and heavy stimulation. Breakfast is a coffee. Mid morning is a coffee. Lunch is barely touched. Dinner is high calorie and unfinished. To this guy, food isn't important, and he's probably just too busy to care that he hardly eats any green foods save for the slice of lettuce on his burger.

THE GUZZLER: Did you know there are 340 calories in a large Caramel Macchiato from Starbucks? This guy doesn't. And, he doesn't care. The guzzler partakes in high calorie drinks such as specialty coffees and sugar-packed sodas and favors beer over wine any day—and partakes almost every day. He eats two or three meals a day but they aren't elaborate or particularly high in fat or calories. Greens aren't on his radar or menu. He's not actively avoiding them, but he won't seek them out either.

THE FAST FILLER: This guy eats out—a lot. And what he does eat out is usually ordered through a microphone and served up in a brown paper bag. Fast food fills out his menu on a very regular basis. If McDonald's has a specialty burger this month, he probably knows about it on the first, and his review is usually favorable. He's probably young and definitely not interested in the nuances of proper nutrition. He eats what he likes, and he doesn't like green foods because he thinks they cost too much, they are too much of a hassle, and he doesn't like the taste.

We've seen these five guys mostly in our years of working with men's fitness, health, and nutrition because these are the guys that need our help. This is not to say that there aren't any vegetarian men, vegans, guys who follow a very regimented and proper diet, or dudes who simply love green foods. They do exist. But science has proven that they are a limited species.

What better proof is there that men don't eat their greens than the fact that scientists have been trying to study the reasons for years? Researchers across the globe have labored over this issue and what they've found is not good. One study conducted in Ohio found that men truly believe that they aren't capable of following a healthy diet. They also found that men don't believe eating a proper diet is all that important to maintaining their health. Another study out of Britain found that men eat fewer vegetables than their infant children. In each case they feel that they have less control over their diet than the women of the house. Further investigation in the study showed that many spouses of the men polled had been trying to remedy the issue by hiding healthier foods in their husbands' diet. Another study furthered this research and offered the conclusion that men simply don't feel eating a healthy diet composed of green foods, lean proteins, vital nutrients, and vitamins is part of their "culture."

The conclusions are all the same. Science, attitudes, and history all agree that men aren't eating their greens. They don't want to change their behavior and have little to no desire to hear why they should. *Green Foods for Men* is an attempt to break that barrier. In our experience, you can't simply tell men what to eat—especially if what you're serving differs from what they crave or have been conditioned to eat. Instead, you have to approach the change with information. Lots of information. You not only have to prove why your method is an improvement, but you also have to prove that your way reflects more than just a few people's opinions. You need hard data, scientific fact, and an approach that allows them to draw their own conclusions. But beyond conclusions, you also need to help them make their own day-to-day decisions. Convince a man to eat healthier and he will, but he won't want you choosing every gram passing his lips. He wants to decide what, how, and how much. And that's exactly why *Green Foods for Men* will work for any man, at any nutritional level, and with any health goal.

This book lists the fifty very best green foods that men can consume. We're not saying you should eat them because they're the tastiest, trendiest, most expensive, or best for the overall population. These foods have a dramatic impact on what matters most to men. Each food entry will show important scientific data for the most vital of male concerns: muscle building, fat loss, improved sex drive, improved appearance, and specific health boosts unique to the male gender. Beyond that, you'll also get the raw caloric and macronutrient information for each food, so you can decide how much is enough. Look out for storage tips, easy-to-follow recipes, and a myriad of options to make each food that much more accessible and realistic for your diet. You'll also find some meal plan challenges. First, for the staunchest opponent of eating green, a three-day challenge that will prove that including green foods in your diet is not only easy, but tasty as hell. Next, a seven-day cleanse uses the power of green foods to make you your best—detoxifying your body and making sure it is firing on every level. And to cap it off, a thirty-day plan will get you on the road to making green foods a part of your life forever.

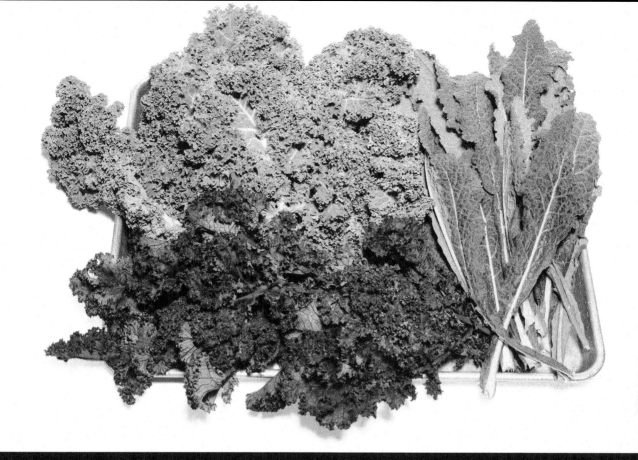

WHY GREEN FOODS WORK

1. EFFICIENT SOURCE OF ENERGY: Even though greens are very low in calories, they help you create energy naturally. First, they are packed with chlorophyll, the component that makes them green. Chlorophyll is the plant's version of blood, transporting oxygen and nutrients throughout the plant, allowing it to grow and thrive. Coincidentally, chlorophyll is similar in structure to your blood cells and can actually help improve how well your blood transports oxygen and nutrients in your body as well.

2. IMPROVED CIRCULATION: The alkaline minerals in the greens improve circulation to deliver the goods to your brain and muscles. You'll notice you won't need to hit the snooze button or have as much coffee to get through your day with the help of greens.

3. RESTOCK YOUR MAGNESIUM: The magnesium in greens is responsible for more than 400 energy pathways in your body, and an estimated 95 percent of us are deficient in this power mineral.

4. REDUCE YOUR TOXINS: These green foods protect you from heavy metal toxicity such as mercury found in sushi or from environmental toxins in urban areas.

5. TO HELP YOUR HANGOVER: Speaking of toxins, greens help your liver by nourishing it with magnesium and oxygen, cleaning up the damage from a booze indulgence or processed foods splurge.

6. TO AGE WITHOUT FEELING LIKE YOU'RE AGING: Methylation is a powerful chemical pathway that aids detoxification. Studies have shown that proper methylation can decrease your risk of cancer, cardiovascular disease, neurological diseases, and other chronic degenerative diseases. If you haven't heard about it yet, you will. An estimated 20 percent of us have a genetic predisposition to being poor methylators. Folate is a superstar methylator, and when you think of folate, think "foliage"… It's in the greens! With the thousands of methyl-dependent reactions going on everyday, you can support them by eating your methylators.

7. TO GET THE MOST OUT OF YOUR FOOD: Raw or lightly sautéed greens contain enzymes that help your digestion so you get the most out of your superfoods. These enzymes help break down the food into their absorbable parts. Plus, the alkaline environment that the greens provide is what is most beneficial when consuming pastured meat and poultry. So, consuming greens with your meal will help you get the most out of it. It's not just what you eat. It's what you digest.

WHEN TO HAVE YOUR GREENS

Ideally you will enjoy green foods in every meal of your day. Because, well, why not have greens at every meal? Don't waste your chance to add greens to every meal or snack you can. Once you make it a habit in every meal, and you happen to have a few unexpected, greenless meals, at least you know your whole day wasn't a big fat zero.

GO-TO GREENS Start developing your list of go-to greens for breakfast, lunch, dinner, snacks, juices, and smoothies. Pick things that you like and challenge yourself to try something new. You might hate Romaine lettuce, but love the flavor of arugula (yes, they taste different). Or, you might avoid cucumbers because you don't want to slice them. There's no excuse with pickles. Once you develop your lineup of green foods, then start adding, guys.

MORE IS BETTER The majority of green foods listed here are not calorically dense, except for pistachios, pumpkin seeds, and avocado. So, don't feel like you have to change up your current portion sizes just to get your greens in. Yes, more is better with green foods.

GREENS FOR BREAKFAST We've found that the hardest time for men to have green foods is in the morning. Whether it's a lack of craving for greens, or a stronger craving for a bowl of Lucky Charms, men aren't reaching for greens until dinnertime, when his significant other insists he eats a salad with dinner. If this is an issue for you, green tea is the least intimidating addition to your morning, followed by green fruits. Then, slowly make your way to adding spinach to your eggs or pistachios to your oatmeal, and finally make the leap to green juices and smoothies to start your day. Having greens for breakfast is a mental hurdle you must get over, or you'll start the day already behind. Who wants that?

GREEN SMOOTHIES 101 Green smoothies are the perfect solution if you hate salads, think eating carrot sticks is lame, or don't like prepping and cooking vegetables. Smoothies were practically designed to win over green food haters. As long as you can get over the green color (or just get some dark cups), green smoothies are sure to please.

Start blending greens, frozen fruit, and a little added natural sweetener such as raw honey. You might start with a more fruit-heavy smoothie, but know that your goal, and where you will see the most benefit, is really in those green vegetables. The hint that you are using enough greens is if your smoothie is actually green in color!

JUICING 101 Juicing fruits and vegetables and including them in your diet is an excellent way to get additional vitamins, minerals, antioxidants, and more in a very easy and delicious way. From a nutrition standpoint, freshly made juices are most beneficial for their quick absorption of nutrients, especially when consumed at least an hour before or after a meal. When juices are consumed with a meal, you are certainly going to obtain those nutrients, but the wow factor of quick absorption and quick energy will not be there since digestion and absorption of these nutrients are not as sudden when paired with a whole meal.

Start juicing fruits and vegetables you are familiar with and already enjoy eating. Carrots and apples are a newbie juicer's best friend and can be a great base as you get going. From there, work on getting more greens. They may not taste great initially, which is why starting with the apple and carrot base is the way to go at first.

That said, your friendliest greens will be celery and cucumber. And your greenest greens will be spinach and kale. Because these juices concentrate the flavor, if you are not a huge fan of spinach taste, then you may need to add more apple. Or, consider smoothies instead, which do not contain as much greens as juices and can better mask the "green" flavor.

EXPERIMENT Use the recipes in this book as templates and adjust the amounts of each ingredient however you see fit. There really is no wrong way to construct a juice. The only caution is to not go overboard on fruit juices, as they will be high in natural sugars, but can be an issue if you have any cravings or potential blood sugar issues. Your goal is to always make sure there is at least one green vegetable in every juice you make.

VARIETY IS KEY Different green foods provide different green benefits. Rotating your go-to greens every few weeks will give you the best results and a variety of nutrients you need.

THE 50 GREEN SUPERFOODS

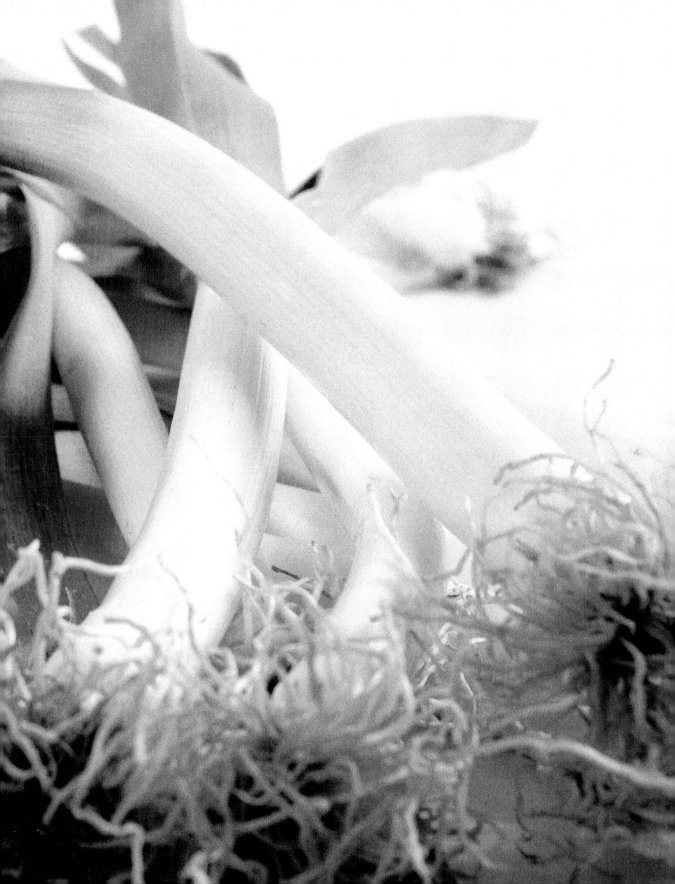

ARTICHOKE

Mother Nature seemingly went to a lot of trouble to prevent you from enjoying all of the goodness in an artichoke. It's the only food in this book that has built-in armor. But you're a big boy and you can get past it— and it'll feel kind of like you hunted and killed this prey. Although it may look more like an organic hand grenade than something you'd like to eat, artichokes are packed with more vital nutrients than almost any other vegetable you've ever shunned at the salad bar.

NUTRITIONAL INFORMATION

1 Artichoke, medium

Calories:	60
Fat:	.19 g
Carbohydrate:	13.45 g
Dietary fiber:	6.9 g
Sugar:	1.27 g
Protein:	4.19 g

YOU NEED TO EAT THIS

MORE NUTRIENTS AND LESS LIVER DAMAGE
Artichokes keep your liver working at optimum levels, which is good for any guy who casually, or frequently, drinks. It also increases the liver's production of bile, which breaks down foods so you can better absorb the nutrients. This means artichokes ensure you get the most out of everything you eat.

STRONGER BONES
What vegetable has the most magnesium and potassium per serving? Artichokes. Why is that important? It builds your bones, making them stronger, leaving you less prone to injuries and way more stable and powerful in any sport or workout.

LIVE LONGER
Packed with flavonoids, polyphenols, and vitamin C, artichokes boost your immune system, help cut the risk of stroke, and lower cholesterol.

BETTER HEALTH
The folate found in artichokes helps reduce inflammation and the risk of heart disease. The roots also help reduce cholesterol.

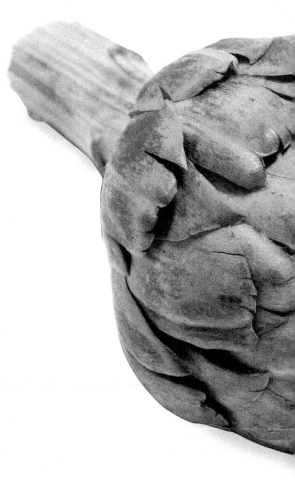

PREP TIPS

- Squeeze it. If it squeaks, it's ready.
- After washing it in cold water, cut one inch (2.5 cm) off the top with a serrated knife, and cut the stem up to a half inch (1.3 cm). The whole stem can be removed if you wish to have the artichoke stand up on its own.
- You can clip the finger nail-like thorns on the leaves, but they do soften when cooked.
- Drizzle with lemon juice to avoid browning while cooking.
- The leaves of the artichoke can also be separated to produce more flavor.
- Most people boil artichokes, but steaming preserves the nutrients. Kick up the flavor by grilling it afterwards.

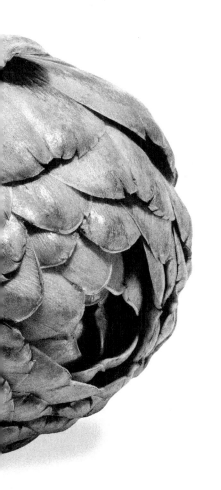

The ★ indicates the estimated servings of green food that this recipe will provide and can guide you in reaching your green food goals during any of the three meal plans.

GARLIC DIJON ARTICHOKES ★ ★

2 fresh artichokes
Water to steam artichokes
½ cup (120 ml) refined coconut oil
1 bulb of garlic, all cloves separated and peeled
¼ cup (44 g) Dijon mustard

Rinse the artichokes thoroughly. Place in a covered pot with 1 inch (2.5 cm) of water at the bottom. Bring water to a boil on high heat. Reduce heat to low and steam, covered, until 2 to 3 outer leaves are easily pulled from each artichoke (20 to 30 minutes or more, depending on size). While the artichokes are steaming, sauté all garlic cloves in coconut oil until tender. Remove artichokes from the water and toss with garlic oil and Dijon mustard.

BASIL ARTICHOKE MEATBALLS ★ ★ ★

½ pound (455 g) ground turkey or grass-fed beef
2 tablespoons (5 g) fresh basil, finely chopped
1 cup (300 g) artichoke hearts, diced
1 tablespoon (15 ml) coconut oil to cook with
Salt and pepper

Place skillet over medium heat and add the coconut oil. Add artichoke hearts and cook for 3 to 4 minutes, then let cool. Once the artichoke hearts have cooled, mix them in a large bowl with the ground meat, basil, salt and pepper. Mix well. Form 2-inch (5 cm) diameter meatballs and place on a baking sheet lined with parchment paper. Bake for 15 to 20 minutes at 350°F (180°C, or gas mark 4) until cooked through.

Easy Add-Ons to Your Diet

1. Add boiled, diced artichokes to eggs and vegetables for a scrambled breakfast.
2. Toss boiled, chilled artichoke leaves into a green salad.
3. Use raw artichoke leaves as chips to dip for hummus or salsa.
4. Roast artichokes and serve with roasted chicken.
5. Add a layer to a lasagna to boost flavor and nutrients.

ARUGULA

Would you skip eating a plant that generations have lauded to give you sexual super powers? Would you pass on green leaves that ancient cultures think give you good luck? If you would, you'd also be missing out on some of the serious benefits of eating arugula, including improving your appearance, health, and sex life. Go ahead and pass on it. There'll be more for the next guy—who's going to be better looking and scooping up your girlfriend. Don't say we didn't warn you.

NUTRITIONAL INFORMATION

1 cup (20 g)

Calories:	6
Fat:	0.2 g
Carbohydrate:	.8 g
Dietary fiber:	.4 g
Sugars:	.4 g
Protein:	.6 g

YOU NEED TO EAT THIS

FAT LOSS

Packed with fiber, this green food isn't just a great alternative to your standard iceberg lettuce. In fact, it helps you metabolize your food more slowly, keeping you fuller longer, so you'll be thinner with every plate.

BETTER SEX

It's been proven that with all of the contaminants in the environment, everything we eat and every breath we take hurts our sex drive. What's also been proven is that arugula and other leafy greats fight off those contaminants and help keep you ready for any bedroom fun.

FULLER HAIR

Some evidence indicates that arugula oil can aid in hair growth. Although more research is needed to see the full extent of this, women have been using oil treatments on their hair for years. So if you're thinning, you might consider adding some arugula oil to the top of your head to help maintain what you've got, strengthen it, and possibly even grow some more.

PREP TIP

• The best way to clean fresh arugula is to submerge it in cold water and swirl it around so any dirt or sand moves to the bottom of the washing basin. Once clean, the leaves can be transferred to a salad spinner to remove excess water. Before cleaning, any yellow-colored or wilted leaves should be removed and stems should be cut.

STORAGE TIP

• You can store arugula in the crisper of your fridge (that's the drawer that you can't see into if you don't know what a crisper is), or you can keep them fresh by leaving them in a cup of water like a plant.

★ = serving of green food

ARUGULA PESTO ★ ★
2 cups (40 g) packed fresh arugula
1 clove garlic
¼ cup (30 g) walnuts
½ cup (120 ml) olive oil
Salt and pepper to taste
Process all of the ingredients in a food processor.
Use in pasta, on meats, or in sandwiches.

ARUGULA-STUFFED TURKEY ROLL UPS ★
2 slices of nitrate-free turkey meat
1 slice uncured, nitrate-free bacon
1 slice avocado
2 slices tomato, raw
½ cup (10 g) arugula
Lay out 2 slices of turkey meat stacked on top of each
other, add bacon, avocado, tomato, and ½ cup (10 g)
arugula onto the turkey slices and roll up tightly.

ARUGULA SALAD ★ ★ ★
2 bunches arugula, washed, dried, and torn
¼ cup (60 ml) extra-virgin olive oil
½ red onion, sliced
½ cup (70 g) toasted pumpkin seeds
½ lemon, juiced
Salt and freshly ground black pepper
In a bowl, toss together the arugula, onions,
and pumpkin seeds. Season with the salt and
pepper. Drizzle with the vinegar and oil and
toss. Taste and re-season if necessary.
Serve immediately.

Easy Add-Ons to Your Diet ~~~~~~~

1. Add very thinly sliced pears, crushed walnuts,
   and lime juice to some arugula for a salad.
2. Use arugula instead of regular lettuce in your
   tacos to add a peppery boost of flavor.
3. Add chopped arugula, diced hot potato, and
   dill to a few scoops of Greek yogurt and mix
   for a fresh potato salad.

ASPARAGUS

Let's discuss the elephant in the room: Yes, asparagus will make your urine smell. There's really not much you can do to prevent that, but including asparagus into a healthy, balanced diet will result in many advantages to counteract that minor nuisance. In fact, this green is more beneficial for you than the steak you're used to seeing it next to simply by supercharging your blood cells. Its nutrients will help you react quicker and build a better you.

YOU NEED TO EAT THIS

FASTER MUSCLE GAINS

Consuming the roots and shoots of asparagus have been proven to help lower high blood pressure and promote greater blood flow. As a result, your body is able to repair quicker after each workout, which will result in faster gains in the gym. Also serving up a high dose of vitamin K, asparagus can help prevent blood clots and cell damage from workouts or any other type of strenuous activity.

FAT LOSS

A great diuretic, including asparagus into your diet can help expel excess water weight and eliminate toxins via increased urine output. Some elite athletes will cut water weight before a weigh in or contest, and asparagus can help for a very short-term weight loss.

BATTLE FRIDAY NIGHT DRINKS

Asparagus leaf extracts have been shown to help safeguard the liver from toxins, including those found in those weekend drinks you share with your pals.

BETTER HEALTH

The folate found in asparagus helps reduce inflammation and the risk of heart disease. The roots also help reduce cholesterol.

STORAGE TIP

• Always refrigerate your asparagus spears. Normally they will last for about three days. Keeping the roots damp in a wet paper towel will help keep them fresh longer.

NUTRITIONAL INFORMATION

1 cup (88 g)

Calories:	27
Fat:	0 g
Carbohydrate:	5 g
Dietary fiber:	3 g
Sugar:	3 g
Protein:	3 g

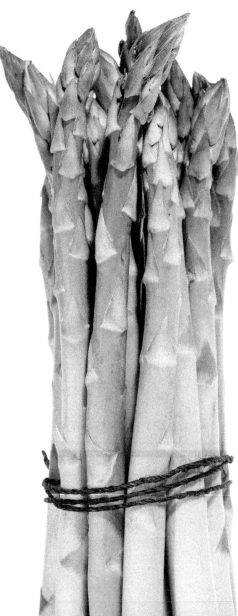

★ = serving of green food

TROPICAL SMOOTHIE ★ ★ ★

7 asparagus spears

2 bananas

2 oranges, peeled

2 cups fresh spinach

1½ cups (220 g) strawberries, fresh or frozen

Blend all ingredients until smooth.

CARROT, ASPARAGUS, TOMATO JUICE ★

10 asparagus spears

12 carrots

1 tomato

Process all of the ingredients through a juicer.

GREEN JUICE ★ ★ ★ ★

2 green apples

1 medium-size cucumber

5 asparagus spears

Process all of the ingredients through a juicer. Green apples are recommended, but red apples give more sweetness.

PROSCIUTTO-WRAPPED ASPARAGUS ★ ★

10 asparagus spears, ¾- to 1-inch (2- to 2.5-cm) thick

1 tablespoon (15 ml) olive oil

Salt and pepper

10 thin slices of prosciutto

Toss the asparagus in the olive oil, salt, and pepper. Wrap each spear with 1 slice of prosciutto in a downward spiral toward the cut end, just barely overlapping the seams of the prosciutto. Place spears on a baking sheet, without touching. Broil for 3 minutes, flip them over, and broil for 3 more minutes.

ASPARAGUS FRITTATA ★ ★

½ cup (44 g) asparagus, chopped

¼ cup (25 g) scallions, chopped

3 eggs

Coconut oil

Sauté vegetables in the coconut oil and let cool in fridge. Add whisked eggs to a greased pan. Add a little water to the eggs to improve fluffiness. Add the cooled vegetables to the pan. Bake at 350°F (180°C or gas mark 4) until eggs are fully cooked (10 to 15 minutes).

PAN-FRIED ASPARAGUS ★

½ stalk asparagus

lemon zest

1 tablespoon (15 ml) coconut oil

Cut asparagus into 4 to 5 inch (10 to 13 cm) long tips. Heat the coconut oil in a frying pan. Add asparagus in a single layer and turn heat to medium-high. Cook the asparagus for 4 to 5 minutes, turning about once a minute. Turn off the heat, then squeeze juice of half the lemon over asparagus. Sprinkle with lemon zest and serve immediately.

Easy Add-Ons to Your Diet ~~~~~~

1. Grill asparagus spears for a charred, smoky addition to your steak.
2. Dice raw asparagus and add it to a salad, tuna sandwich, or even your guacamole.
3. Puree it in a blender and mix with milk or coconut milk and chicken broth and simmer for a five-minute soup.
4. Add it to a stir fry with other vegetables and protein of your choice.
5. Roast it in the oven with a light sprinkling of pepper flakes and Parmesan for a side dish or snack.

AVOCADO

Sometimes referred to as the alligator pear, the avocado fruit is native to central Mexico. Most guys consider avocado to be nothing more than the backbone of the guacamole that starts off a night of watching the big game, but this green superfood is much more than just an ingredient in a popular dip. In fact, a 2013 study revealed that avocado eaters in the United States had a better overall diet and a reduced risk of cardiovascular disease and diabetes. Moreover, it packs a serious punch at heart disease, gastritis, and high cholesterol.

NUTRITIONAL INFORMATION

½ avocado

Calories:	114
Fat:	11 g
Carbohydrate:	6 g
Dietary fiber:	4.5 g
Sugar:	0 g
Protein:	1.5 g

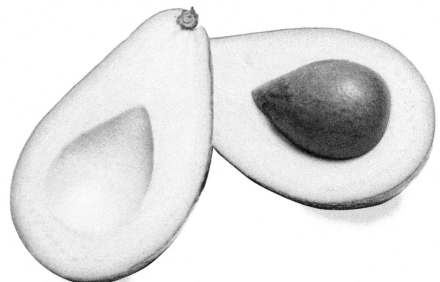

YOU NEED TO EAT THIS

FOR BETTER SEXUAL PERFORMANCE

Avocado contains essential fatty acids needed for male hormone production, including testosterone, as well as phytochemicals and three powerful antioxidants: vitamin C, vitamin E, and glutathione—all of which work to improve sexual function.

INCREASE ENERGY LEVELS

An excellent source of folate, with 118.26 µg per serving—which is 29.6 percent of the recommended daily intake—avocados help convert fats, proteins, and carbohydrates into energy.

BUILD MUSCLE

One serving of avocado has 152 µg of potassium, or 4 percent of the recommended daily intake value for men, which is essential for protein synthesis—the foundation of building muscle.

IMPROVE YOUR CHANCES OF CONCEIVING

Some preliminary research shows that combining green foods like avocado with celery on a daily basis can improve sperm count. Why? Foods with folate (avocado) and zinc (celery) work together to increase sperm motility.

★ = serving of green food

GUACAMOLE ★

2 avocados

1 cup (260 g) salsa

1 teaspoon (5 ml) lemon juice

Salt and pepper to taste

Mash avocados with a fork. Stir in the salsa, lemon juice, and salt/pepper. For a spice kick, add finely diced jalapenos.

AVOCADO PUDDING ★ ★ ★

1 ripe avocado

½ cup (120 ml) unsweetened coconut milk

1 tablespoon (20 g) raw honey

2 tablespoons (18 g) pistachios, crushed

Blend ingredients by hand or in a food processor, until smooth. Serve chilled. Sprinkle with the pistachios.

WAFFLE BREAKFAST SANDWICH ★

2 eggs

2 teaspoons (10 ml) coconut oil

2 slices avocado

2 gluten free waffles

2 ounces (55 g) bacon or pork sausage patty, no nitrates added

1 tablespoon (20 ml) organic maple syrup

Fry 2 to 3 eggs in the coconut oil. Place them on a gluten-free waffle. Add two slices of avocado, a slice of no nitrate-added bacon, and drizzle with organic maple syrup. Then, place another waffle on top to complete the sandwich. **OPTIONAL:** Spread the waffle with pesto sauce for a sweet savory combination of flavors.

AVOCADO CHICKEN SALAD ★ ★ ★

2 boneless, skinless chicken breasts

½ avocado

¼ onion, chopped

Juice of ½ lime

2 tablespoons (5 g) fresh chopped cilantro or basil

Cook the chicken breasts until done; let them cool and then shred. Add the avocado and onion and mix. Add the lime juice and a few tablespoons of the cilantro or basil for added flavor.

AVOCADO VINAIGRETTE ★ ★ ★ ★

BY CHEF JOSH KATT, OWNER OF KITCHFIX

1 avocado, ripe

1 lime, juiced

1 tablespoon (2.5 g) cilantro, chopped

1 tablespoon (15 ml) water

Salt and pepper to taste

A pinch of cumin

Cut the avocado in half; remove the seed carefully; and scoop the flesh from the skin into a bowl. Cut the lime in half, and squeeze it over the avocado. Add the chopped cilantro, a pinch of cumin, and the salt and pepper to taste. Finally add the water, and start to mash and mix the avocado until smooth.

STORAGE TIP

• Store unripe avocados in paper bags and they will ripen quicker. Splash lemon or lime juice onto the unused portion of an avocado to stave off the browning of the fruit.

IS IT READY?
PEEL OFF THE LITTLE STEM ON THE BOTTOM OF THE AVOCADO TO SEE IF IT IS GREEN AND THEREFORE RIPE.

Easy Add-Ons to Your Diet

1. Add avocado to a smoothie to increase the creaminess and stabilize blood sugar for sustaining energy.
2. Add mashed avocado in place of mayonnaise, butter, cheese, sour cream, or other dairy-based spreads.
3. While it seems like an unusual combination, avocados actually make a fantastic creamy pasta sauce, too. Combined with lemon, garlic, olive oil, Parmesan cheese, and basil, it's like a healthier (and greener) version of the classic Alfredo sauce. Add some extra green veggies to the mix to make it even healthier.

BASIL

If you think that basil is just the green bits you see in your pasta sauce, you're dead wrong. Every culture since the dawn of time has found a plethora of uses for basil, and we don't mean as garnish on your plate! In fact, basil could possibly be the most versatile food in this book because it can be used in virtually any meal, snack, or drink. And versatility isn't its only plus; it's also bringing more health benefits to the table than just about anything else you've eaten this week.

NUTRITIONAL INFORMATION

2 tablespoons (5 g), fresh

Calories:	1
Fat:	0 g
Carbohydrate:	0.1 g
Dietary fiber:	0.1 g
Sugar:	0 g
Protein:	0.2 g

YOU NEED TO EAT THIS

STAY YOUNG
Basil has a specific anti-aging quality, especially for your liver, brain, and heart. It also helps your kidneys expel toxins and promotes overall better health.

MORE MUSCLE
Two tablespoons (5 g) of fresh basil has only 1 calorie, but surprisingly it contains anywhere from 60 to 70 percent of the daily value for vitamin K. It also assists in the regulation of blood flow, thus allowing your body to repair and promote more muscle gains. Want more? It's vital to the blood clotting process, meaning that without proper levels of it in your system, you could die.

KILL BACTERIA
Essential oil of basil has been shown to kill antibiotic resistant strains of bacteria, so you can consider this a worthy adversary in the battle against all the superbugs popping up. In fact, just coming into contact with basil can fend off the bacteria found on other produce, which means consuming this green will ensure you get everything you need and nothing you don't from what you're eating.

Easy Add-Ons to Your Diet

1. Mix into raw ground meats before shaping burgers, meatballs, or meatloaf.
2. Add to plain water for a unique thirst quencher that will also freshen your breath and help detoxify your system.

★ = serving of green food

WATERMELON AND BASIL SALAD ★ ★ ★ ★
2 cups (300 g) watermelon, cubed
2 tablespoons (5 g) basil
Juice and zest of 1 lime
1 tablespoon (15 ml) olive oil
¼ cup (34 g) chopped jalapeños
Put the watermelon cubes in a bowl. Whisk together the lime juice, zest, olive oil, and chopped jalapeño. Pour this over the watermelon and toss to combine. Cover and refrigerate for 30 minutes and then serve.

COOKING TIPS
• Add basil to your dish last so it retains its potency.
• Also, the thicker the stem, the more bitter the flavor—cooked or raw.

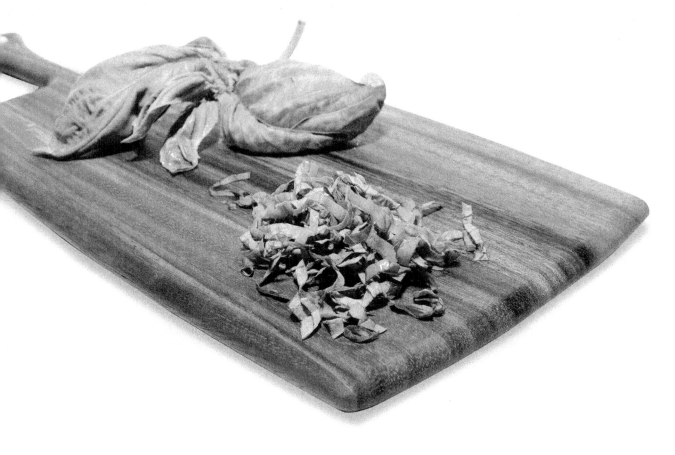

TASTES

BASIL AVOCADO SAUCE ★ ★ ★ ★

¾ cup (30 g) fresh basil leaves (stems removed)

1 small avocado (pits and skin removed)

1 tablespoon (15 ml) of extra-virgin olive oil

Dash of salt and ground black pepper

Place the basil, avocado, olive oil, salt, and ground black pepper in a food processor and blend until smooth.
Use on grilled chicken/fish, on tacos, or as pasta sauce.

BASIL VINAIGRETTE ★ ★

2 cups (80 g) basil leaves

½ cup (120 ml) olive oil

¼ cup (60 ml) white wine or champagne vinegar

1 small clove garlic

Salt and pepper to taste

In a blender or food processor, blend the basil, oil, vinegar, and garlic until smooth. Add salt and pepper to taste.

BASIL-INFUSED BRUSCHETTA ★ ★

¼ cup (60 ml) extra-virgin olive oil

7 basil leaves, chopped

1½ pounds (680 g) plum tomatoes, diced

2 cloves garlic, minced

1 French baguette, sliced

Toss together ingredients. Serve on toasted baguette slices.

STRAWBERRY BASIL CHICKEN ★ ★

4 to 6 ounces (115 to 165 g) chicken breast, pasture raised

½ cup (75 g) strawberries, sliced

3 tablespoons (45 ml) balsamic vinegar

2 tablespoons (5 g) basil, chopped

1 cup (30 g) spinach, sauteed

Combine the strawberries, balsamic vinegar, and basil. Serve on top of sautéed spinach and pasture-raised grilled chicken.

BEET GREENS

Beet greens are considered a wild plant and are actually more impressive nutritionally than the beet root you've been avoiding at the salad bar (also known as the red part most people serve). Early Romans only ate the beet greens, and left the beet roots for medicinal purposes. These days, research has shown that these greens can help fight cancer, improve your vision, and make your bones stronger.

NUTRITIONAL INFORMATION

1 cup (225 g)

Calories:	8
Fat:	.05 g
Carbohydrate:	1.65 g
Dietary fiber:	1.4 g
Sugar:	.19 g
Protein:	.84 g

YOU NEED TO EAT THIS

BETTER PERFORMANCE

Beet greens improve the transport of oxygen to the blood and muscles. That means you'll be better in the gym, on the court, and in the sack.

BETTER SKIN, HEALTHIER HAIR, AND BETTER VISION

Packed with vitamin A, beet greens can help improve your skin, helping you look younger and healthier. It's also your secret weapon against hyperkeratosis, which is the accumulation of clumps of dry skin around your hair follicles. Vitamin A is also essential for the retina to transform light, so it's vital for vision. As a matter of fact, if you've ever had a bout of night blindness, your doctor has probably already put you on a vitamin A supplement.

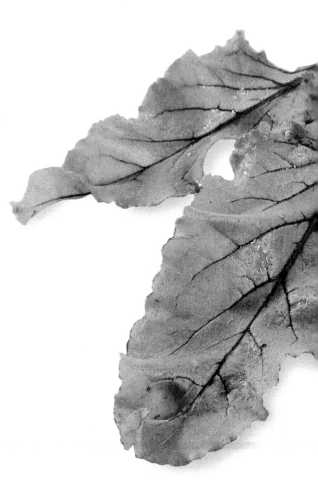

★ = serving of green food

BANANA AND BEET GREEN SMOOTHIE ★

1 cup (235 ml) water

1 cup (225 g) beet greens, chopped, thick stems removed

1 fresh or frozen banana

1 tablespoon (20 g) raw honey or Grade B maple syrup to sweeten (optional)

Blend all of the ingredients until smooth.

Easy Add-Ons to Your Diet

1. Chop up and add to a salad, stir fry, sandwich, or taco.
2. Add to your juicing mixes for a powerful antioxidant punch.
3. Freeze and use them later as stock for a soup.

COOKING TIPS

• Make sure the greens you're using aren't yellowed and have no brown spots.

• Look for a tight leaf with sturdy stems, chop according to desired size after cleaning and add to salads.

• You can also boil or sauté your beet greens, making sure to add olive oil and sea salt for extra flavor.

BOK CHOY

Sounds more like a bad chicken impersonation than a vegetable, right? Don't sweat it. Once you get past the name, this super green will amaze you. Ready to be amazed? Okay, first off, chances are you've already eaten bok choy and you didn't even know it! Found in most Chinese takeout, bok choy is a staple of many Asian dishes. Why? Well maybe it's the outstanding hearty flavor or the fact that it could save your life. Sound like good enough reasons for you to incorporate it into your meal plan?

NUTRITIONAL INFORMATION

1 cup (70 g), shredded

Calories:	9
Fat:	.02 g
Carbohydrate:	1.53 g
Dietary fiber:	.7 g
Sugar:	.83 g
Protein:	4.19 g

YOU NEED TO EAT THIS

STRONG BONES

Packed with calcium, bok choy can be an alternative for maintaining strong bones, especially for those avoiding dairy.

LOWER BLOOD PRESSURE

Got high blood pressure? Bok choy can help. The high potassium content in this green vegetable regulates your muscles and blood flow while simultaneously lowering your blood pressure levels.

FIGHT CANCER

This simple plant is loaded with so many nutrients, it's hard not to list it as a cure-all. We think you'll agree after we've told you that it can help reduce the risk of bladder and lung cancers. Ready to call it a superfood yet?

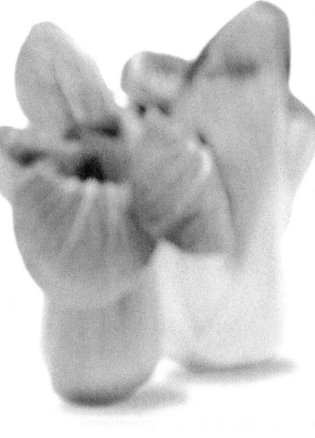

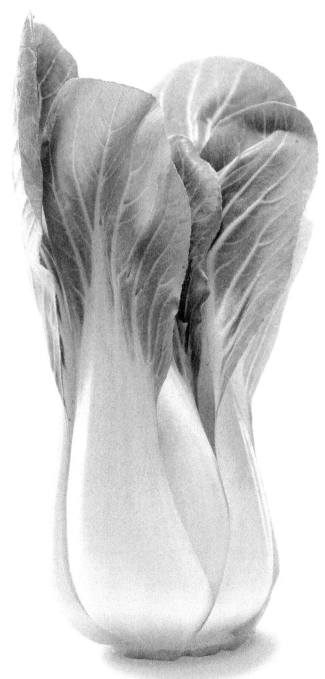

★ = serving of green food

ASIAN STIR FRY ★ ★ ★ ★
4 to 6 ounces (115 to 170 g) of chicken or steak,
   cut into small pieces
½ cup (75 g) green bell peppers, chopped
½ cup (35 g) broccoli, chopped
1 cup (70 g) bok choy, chopped
1 tablespoon (15 ml) coconut aminos
1 tablespoon (15 ml) coconut oil

Cook the meat in a pan using the coconut oil.
Remove the meat. Next, sauté the vegetables in the
same pan. Then add the coconut aminos and meat at
the end of cooking.

Easy Add-Ons to Your Diet

1. Chop up and add to a salad or stir fry.
2. Shred and add to your coleslaw mix.
3. Use as stock in a soup—it means "soup
   spoon" in Chinese for a reason.

COOKING TIPS

• Baby bok choy can be eaten whole or cut
in halves or quarters, but bok choy needs
further care.
• Any tough leaves should be removed from the
bunch, and the base of the stalk should be cut off.
• The bok choy leaves should be torn off the stalk
and the leaves should be washed in cold water
before cooking.
• An easy way to clean any dirt or grit on the
leaves is to rub the leaves together when you
are washing them.
• If you plan to sauté the leaves, start cooking the
stems first, which take longer to cook.

BROCCOLI

You probably hate broccoli. It's okay; you can admit it. We understand. How many of us were served up awful bowls full of this sloppy, boiled, rubbery, plant-like substance? Too many of us. But, things change, and we've learned that broccoli not only tastes better raw, it's actually better for you to consume in this manner as well—three times better as a matter of fact. It has more vitamin C than an orange, more calcium than whole milk, and it fights cancer. It's kind of a big deal, and it's time to forgive broccoli and give it another chance.

NUTRITIONAL INFORMATION

1 cup (71 g), raw

Calories:	31
Fat:	.34 g
Carbohydrate:	6.04 g
Dietary fiber:	2.4 g
Sugar:	1.55 g
Protein:	2.57 g

YOU NEED TO EAT THIS

BEAT CANCER

Broccoli, more than just about any other thing you can eat, is a cancer-fighting ninja. There's no other way to look at it. In fact, two servings of broccoli, or other cruciferous veggies, per day reduces anyone's risk of cancer by 50 percent—so share it with your wife. But when you combine broccoli with tomatoes, they work together to specifically reduce prostate tumors—so make sure you get more than enough for yourself! No wonder broccoli consumption has gone up 900 percent in the last twenty-five years.

BETTER BLOOD, HEALTHIER YOU

When you're serving up vitamin C, E, quercetin, laempferol, glucosinolates, and glucoraphanin like broccoli does, you're hardwired to blast away cancer-causing chemical carcinogens and harmful free radicals from the body. You also outright kill cancer cells and decrease inflammation. All of this makes you a whole lot healthier, inside and out.

HEALTHIER LOOKING SKIN

Women are always looking for ways to get rid of wrinkles. Now, you know a simple solution—go ahead and share it, if you want to be a nice guy. Broccoli—specifically the sprouts—is packed with sulforaphane, which has been proven to help your skin look its best.

PREP TIPS

- Organic broccoli has more phytonutrients than non-organic fare.
- If it's yellow, it is past its prime. The smaller the broccoli head, the better the flavor.
- Never wash before refrigerating.
- Microwaving and boiling will drastically reduce the nutritional value of your servings. Blanching or steaming is the best cooking method.

★ = serving of green food

BROCCOLI JUICE ★ ★ ★ ★ ★ ★

4 cups (284 g) broccoli

1 cucumber

1 lemon (peeled)

1 large, ripe pear

Process all of the ingredients through a juicer. Serve cold.

BEEF & BROCCOLI STIR FRY ★ ★ ★ ★

4 to 6 ounces (115 to 170 g) grass-fed steak

1 to 2 tablespoons (15 to 30 ml) refined coconut oil

1 tablespoon (8 g) grated fresh ginger

2 cups (142 g) broccoli, chopped

Cook beef pieces in the coconut oil. Remove cooked meat from the pan. Add the broccoli. Cook the broccoli for 2 to 3 minutes. Add the grated ginger to the broccoli and continue cooking until broccoli is fork tender.

GREENS, EGGS, AND HAM ★ ★ ★ ★

Coconut oil

2 eggs

¼ cup (40 g) green onions, chopped

½ cup (35 g) kale, chopped

¼ cup (18 g) broccoli, chopped

2 ounces (55 g) ham, chopped

2 slices avocado

½ cup (15 g) spinach

Coat a frying pan in coconut oil. Add 2 whisked eggs and 2 tablespoons (30 ml) of water. Add the chopped green onions, kale, and finely chopped broccoli. Finally, add the chopped ham. Serve on a bed of spinach and garnish with sliced avocado.

Easy Add-Ons to Your Diet ～～～～

1. Mince and add to scrambled eggs, salads, spreads, or stir fry.
2. Dice and add to wraps, tacos, or burritos.
3. Add to rice or soups for a crunch and nutritional boost.

BRUSSELS SPROUTS

Call Brussels sprouts whatever you want: bone builder, flu killer, power booster, cancer fighter, and all-around superfood, but what you should call it is the key to living longer, creating life, and living your life to its fullest. Love it or hate it (and let's face it: You probably hate it), these little green guys should be in your diet.

NUTRITIONAL INFORMATION

1 cup (88 g)

Calories:	38
Fat:	0.3 g
Carbohydrate:	8 g
Dietary fiber:	3.3 g
Sugar:	1.9 g
Protein:	3 g

YOU NEED TO EAT THIS

LIVE LONGER

Atherosclerosis is your enemy. It raises blood pressure, reduces the elasticity of your arteries, and allows less blood to travel around your body. If you're a healthy, active, gym-going, sport-playing weekend warrior, this is going to really put pressure on your heart. If you're not the most active guy, this could just kill you. The bottom line is that Brussels sprouts can be your secret weapon against atherosclerosis and it can help you live longer and have a healthier heart.

GET HER PREGNANT

If you've been trying to have kids with your significant other and haven't seen any results, you should throw some Brussels sprouts into your diet. It increases your sperm levels and helps prepare her womb for conception. It'll boost fertility in both you and your partner and reduce the risk of miscarriages and birth defects.

LOSE WEIGHT

Packed with fiber, this vegetable won't just keep you regular, help promote colon health, and give you a decent protein punch, it will also fill you up at the dinner table. Eating Brussels sprouts will help you stay fuller longer by keeping energy and blood sugar stable.

BUYING TIPS

• Unless you're shopping at a really high-end shop, you're probably not going to find Brussels sprouts on the stem like those pictured here. What you will find are an assortment of little green balls the size of a big gumball.
• Look for a bright green color and tightly packed leaves.
• If you do get them on the stem, store it all together in water to keep them fresh—pulling off the ones you want when you need them.
• If you're buying them off the vine, store them in a plastic bag in your crisper—they'll keep for seven to ten days.

★ = serving of green food

BRUSSELS SPROUTS SALAD ★ ★ ★ ★ ★ ★

1 green apple, chopped

2 cups (176 g) raw Brussels sprouts, shredded

3 tablespoons (45 ml) apple cider vinegar

2 tablespoons (40 g) raw honey

¼ cup (59 ml) olive oil

Salt and freshly ground black pepper

Combine apple cider vinegar, honey, and olive oil in a container and mix well. Pour it over the apple and Brussels sprouts. Chill in fridge 2 hours before serving. Add salt and ground black pepper to taste.

BACON BALSAMIC BRUSSELS SPROUTS ★ ★ ★ ★

2 cups (176 g) Brussels sprouts

4 ounces (115 g) bacon (nitrate free)

2 onions, sliced

1 tablespoon (20 g) Grade B maple syrup

1 tablespoon (15 ml) balsamic vinegar

Coconut oil

Chop bacon into small pieces and sauté in the coconut oil until brown. Chop onion and add it to the pan and sauté for a few minutes. Add the Brussels sprouts and balsamic vinegar, adding water if it gets too sticky. Cook until tender and drizzle with the maple syrup.

Easy Add-Ons to Your Diet

1. Sauté with chopped bacon and onions.
2. Grate over a saucy dish or into a soup.
3. Grill until there is browning on the edges of the outside leaves; shave some Parmesan on top and enjoy.
4. Add raw Brussels sprouts to your morning smoothie.

CELERY

Let's face it: It's easy to look at celery as a delivery mechanism for peanut butter or something you slice up to add crunch to a tuna salad sandwich. But this simple vegetable has been proven to help prevent various cardiovascular diseases. Celery is also considered a negative calorie food because the act of chewing it burns more calories than you consume.

NUTRITIONAL INFORMATION

2 medium stalks

Calories:	12
Fat:	0.2 g
Carbohydrate:	2.4 g
Dietary fiber:	1.2 g
Sugar:	1.4 g
Protein:	.6 g

YOU NEED TO EAT THIS

FOR BETTER ERECTIONS
Packed with phytonutrients, one of the most important compounds found in celery is a substance called phthalides, which allows celery to act as a vasodilator, a process that helps men experience better erections.

AS A NATURAL PHEROMONE
Some studies suggest that consuming androsterone, which is found in celery cytoplasm, can increase libido in women. If it helps her mood towards you, then the nutritional grand slam it additionally brings to the table (rich sources of carotene, ascorbic acid, riboflavin, folic acid, calcium, iron, and phosphorus) will ensure you're at your best on every level!

FOR HYDRATION
Celery is composed of more than 90 percent water. Because of this, celery is a hydration all-star and is perfect for hydrating throughout the day, pre- and post-workout and during rigorous exercise.

FOR FAT LOSS
A staple of many diets, celery is the perfect vegetable to include in any weight-loss strategy because of its high levels of water and its ability to fill the stomach on fewer calories. Celery also has a very high level of calcium, a proven factor in helping to reduce fat and weight gain for men.

STORAGE TIPS
• Always store celery in cool temperatures, as warm temperatures will cause the high water content to evaporate.
• If your celery is wilted, you can restore some of its crispness by refrigerating it in a container of water.

☆ = serving of green food

CELERY SLAW ☆ ☆ ☆ ☆ ☆ ☆ ☆

4 stalks celery, finely chopped
½ head of cabbage, shredded
½ medium cucumber, finely chopped
⅓ cup (78 ml) extra-virgin olive oil
Juice from two limes
1 clove of garlic, crushed

Combine the cabbage, celery, and cucumber in a bowl. Whisk the oil, lime juice, and garlic. Then pour onto vegetables and mix.

SAUTÉED CELERY ☆ ☆ ☆ ☆ ☆

6 stalks celery
1 bunch of green onion
1 teaspoon (5 ml) extra-virgin olive oil

First, slice or chop the celery stalks. Place a frying pan with a lid over medium heat and add 1 teaspoon (5 ml) of extra-virgin olive oil. When the liquid is hot, add the celery. Cook until crisp tender, about 5 minutes. Add chopped green onion and serve.

AB AND VEG ☆

Carrots and celery with almond butter

PROTEIN SALAD ☆ ☆ ☆ ☆ ☆ ☆

1 can (6½ ounces (185 g)) tuna, drained and flaked
½ cup (50 g) green beans
½ cup (85 g) lima beans
½ cup (50 g) chopped celery
3 cups (70 g) arugula
3 dried leafs of oregano, flaked
¼ cup (60 g) Greek yogurt
Juice from half a lime

Combine the first six ingredients in a small bowl and mix. Whisk yogurt with the lime juice and oregano. Then, pour into mixture. Mix and serve.

APPLE CELERY JUICE ☆ ☆

1 green apple
6 celery stalks

Process all of the ingredients through a juicer. Serve cold.

REAL GREEN JUICE ☆ ☆ ☆ ☆ ☆

2 cups (60 g) spinach
4 celery stalks
2 cups (135 g) kale
1 medium apple, cored
1 large cucumber

Process all of the ingredients through a juicer. Serve cold.

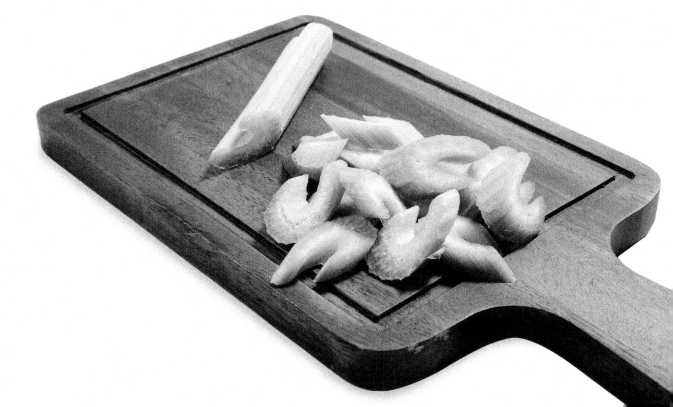

CILANTRO

Many people hate cilantro. There are even entire websites devoted to this simple fact. No doubt many of the folks who made those sites are men. If you've never taken a steak knife and used it to flick a piece of cilantro off a steak to get to the real meal, then you're probably not a guy. But sometimes you've got to eat things you may not love and cilantro is definitely one of them. Bottom line: It'll keep you healthy and help with your post-workout pains among many other benefits.

NUTRITIONAL INFORMATION

¼ cup fresh (4 g)

Calories:	1
Fat:	.02 g
Carbohydrate:	.15 g
Dietary fiber:	.1 g
Sugar:	.03 g
Protein:	.09 g

YOU NEED TO EAT THIS

BEAT MUSCLE PAIN

Hitting the gym hard is as manly as fast cars and football. The soreness that comes thereafter is a tolerated side effect. Throwing some cilantro into your diet could relieve some of that soreness. In fact, cilantro has been proven to be such a good anti-inflammatory that it can also help older adults with arthritic pain.

STAY HEALTHY

Cilantro kicks harmful metals like mercury out of your system while also helping remove harmful toxic contaminants, making you a pre-emptive healthy machine. It also contains an antibiotic called dodecenal known as a salmonella killer.

PROTECT YOUR GUT

Stomach problems? No sweat. Cilantro leaves and seeds help with digestion and distention and relieve intestinal gas and pain. It's also loaded with fiber, which will keep you fuller longer while also helping flush out your system.

★ = serving of green food

CREAMY CILANTRO SAUCE ★ ★ ★ ★
1 cup (16 g) chopped cilantro
½ cup (30 g) chopped parsley
½ cup (60 g) walnuts
¼ cup (60 ml) olive oil
½ medium orange, juiced
1 tablespoon (15 ml) apple cider vinegar
2 tablespoons (30 ml) water
1 teaspoon (0.7 g) fresh rosemary, chopped
Salt and pepper to taste
Blend in a food processor. Use on grilled chicken/fish, on tacos, or as a pasta sauce.

CILANTRO SMOOTHIE ★ ★ ★
1½ cups (45 g) spinach, fresh
½ cup (8 g) cilantro, fresh
1½ cups (250 g) mango
2 cups (475 ml) water
1 cup (165 g) pineapple
½ avocado
Blend until smooth. Enjoy immediately.

CILANTRO CAULIFLOWER RICE ★ ★
2 cups (200 g) cauliflower, roughly chopped
½ lime, juiced
3 tablespoons (3 g) cilantro, fresh and chopped
Use a food processor to grate the cauliflower so it is about rice size, and not completely pulverized. Add the lemon juice and cilantro and serve.

AVOCADO-CILANTRO RICE ★ ★ ★
2 cups (320 g) quick cooking brown rice
1 avocado, mashed
Zest and juice of 1 lime
1 teaspoon (5 g) salt
¼ cup (4 g) fresh cilantro, chopped
Cook rice based on package instructions. Mash avocado and combine with lime juice, lime zest, salt, and cilantro. Combine with rice. Makes two servings.

Easy Add-Ons to Your Diet ～～～～

1. Add leaves to any protein source.
2. Include it in your green salads, potato salads, rice, or any soup.
3. Add to dips and salsas.

STORAGE TIPS

• To prepare for storage, pick out all of the wilted leaves, but keep the roots attached as they can last up to one week while leaves alone only last about three days. Place the bunch with the roots in a jar filled with water. The leaves should then be covered with a loosely fitting plastic bag and the jar should be stored in the refrigerator. For best results, replace the water every couple of days and throw out any wilted leaves. If the roots have already been removed, then use a damp paper towel or cloth to wrap around the leaves and put them in a plastic bag to store in the refrigerator.

• If cilantro is stored frozen, it can be placed in airtight containers either whole or chopped. To maintain the texture, it should never be thawed. Another storage option is to freeze the cilantro with water or stock in ice cube trays, which can then be used for cooking stews or soups.

COLLARD GREENS

If you're from the South, collard greens have probably been on your plate more than a few times. The problem with what you've eaten in the past is that the preparation was filled with a little too much Southern comfort to be healthy. If you've never eaten collard greens, then you're in the same boat as your brothers to the south on this one because we're suggesting you eat them clean: Use the raw leaves in wraps or salads, or eat the cooked varieties with a healthier fat, such as coconut oil, to help it down your throat. Think you can handle it? Well, you might just live a lot longer if you do.

NUTRITIONAL INFORMATION

1 cup (30 g), chopped

Calories:	12
Fat:	.22 g
Carbohydrate:	1.95 g
Dietary fiber:	1.4 g
Sugar:	.17 g
Protein:	1.09 g

YOU NEED TO EAT THIS

BE MORE FERTILE

If you think that oysters are your only source of boosting your sexual super-powers, then your partner probably won't be getting pregnant anytime soon. A diet full of nutrient-dense vitamins and minerals found in collard greens has been proven to help protect your sperm from cellular damage and make your swimmers faster than Michael Phelps in an Olympic pool.

BLAST FAT

Why starve yourself? The simplest way to look at weight loss is that you need to fill your gut with the right stuff so your body can burn off the excess. Ultimately, that means eating low calorie meals, not necessarily eating less. Pack your stomach full of low calorie foods like collard greens. You'll be full and your body will be burning off all the cheeseburgers of the past.

STRONGER BONES

One cup (30 g) of collard greens has more bone-building calcium than a cup of milk. Add in some vitamin C, and your body is almost guaranteed to absorb all that calcium in record time. Also, collard greens are high in vitamin K, which will take your calcium-laced bones and make them even stronger. That means fewer injuries, a stronger frame for building more muscle, and quite possibly winning your local bar's arm wrestling challenge.

BUYING TIPS

• Firm collard green leaves are on your shopping list. Make sure there is no wilting on the leaf and that your grocer has been storing them in a refrigerated state. If they're yellow or brown, pass on them.
• Smaller leaves are younger and less bitter.
• When you get them home, keep them refrigerated in a plastic bag that's sealed with as little air inside as possible.

★ = serving of green food

SAUTÉED LEMON GARLIC COLLARD GREENS ★ ★

2 cups (60 g) collard greens

Pinch or two of salt

Lemon juice

2 teaspoons (10 g) garlic

Boil the collard greens for 3 minutes in salt water. Drain in a colander and then immerse the greens in a bowl of cold water to stop the cooking process. Gather a handful of greens, lift them out of the water, and squeeze dry. Chop the leaves, sauté them in coconut oil, and add lemon and garlic for flavor.

ENERGY-PACKED GREENS ★ ★ ★ ★

BY CHEF JOSH KATT, OWNER OF KITCHFIX

4 cups (275 g) leafy greens, roughly chopped (kale, collard greens, or spinach)

½ an apple, sliced thin

½ an onion, julienned (cut in half, then sliced)

1 tablespoon (15 ml) coconut oil

1 small clove garlic, minced

Salt and pepper to taste

Heat a large pan over medium high heat and add the coconut oil to melt. Once the oil is hot, add the julienned onion and sauté. As the onions start to brown, add the thinly sliced apples. After stirring the apples and onions around together, season them with a touch of salt and pepper. If adding garlic, add at this point. The pan should be sizzling as you're stirring the ingredients around. Add the greens. At first the pan will be overwhelmed, but very quickly the greens will start to lose their water and dramatically decrease in size. Keep stirring. Once the greens have cooked for 3 to 4 minutes remove them from the pan and serve. **TIP:** Make sure to cut your greens small so they are easy to eat later. This dish works great with pork or chicken.

STUFFED COLLARD GREENS ★ ★ ★ ★

3 collard green leaves, blanched

½ head green cabbage, chopped

8 Brussels sprouts, finely chopped

5 asparagus stalks, chopped

1 small sweet potato, finely diced

½ cup (86 g) cooked quinoa

Lightly stir fry collard greens in the coconut oil until wilted. Place the chopped vegetables, potato, and quinoa into the center of a collard green and wrap. Place the wraps into a baking dish. Bake at 350°F (180°C or gas mark 4) for 40 minutes.

Easy Add-Ons to Your Diet ~~~

1. Use leaves as wraps for sandwiches, dropping the bread slices and subsequent carbs.
2. Wrap ground meats in the leaves to make a green taco.

CUCUMBER

Cucumber has probably been in your diet since you were a kid. They're common, they're plentiful, and they're easily bypassed. We're suggesting that you go back to the cucumber dish and pick up more than just a couple slices. It'll help you grow hair, stay hydrated, and help you look better than you've ever thought possible.

NUTRITIONAL INFORMATION

½ cup (60 g) slices

Calories:	8
Fat:	0 g
Carbohydrate:	1.89 g
Dietary fiber:	0.3 g
Sugar:	0.87 g
Protein:	0.34 g

YOU NEED TO EAT THIS

GROW MORE HAIR

Getting a little thin on the top there, buddy? What if we told you that instead of putting harmful chemicals on your scalp, all you had to do was eat something that's been in your diet since you were a little kid? Interested? We thought so. Cucumber is your super-friend for hair growth. Packed with silica, which is an important element to your hair, cucumber will not only help prevent baldness, it can also stimulate new hair growth.

STAY HYDRATED

Why is cucumber an excellent food to help you stay hydrated? It's composed of 95 percent water. Simple enough for you?

BETTER SKIN

With magnesium, silicon, and potassium in its delivery dossier, cucumbers become a skin-improving shaman for all guys out there. Did you think women were putting them on their eyes just to avoid looking at you? It also has a bio-available form of silica that can help heal damage to your skin, nails, and hair.

★ = serving of green food

NATURE'S JUST FOR MEN JUICE ★ ★

½ pineapple, chopped

2 small cucumbers

1 inch (2.5 cm) piece of ginger

Process all of the ingredients through a juicer. Serve cold.

CUCUMBER WATER ★

Slice a cucumber and add it to water. Make sure to wash well before adding, if keeping the peel on.

Easy Add-Ons to Your Diet

1. Use in salads, sandwiches, and wraps.
2. Slice and drizzle with lime juice after sprinkling some paprika on top for a fresh snack with some kick.
3. Replace chips with cucumber slices for dip dishes such as guacamole, salsa, or artichoke dip.
4. Add sliced cucumber to your water for a boost in fresh flavor.

STORAGE TIPS

• Refrigeration is all you really need to do to keep this one lasting for about a week.

• If you cut a cucumber, don't store it past a couple of days.

DILL

You've encountered dill in your past. It's probably been on a plate of fish and you've eaten it without paying any real attention to it. If you've looked into it any further, you probably think it's bunk because so many people out there are saying so many amazing things about how dill can improve your health. It's not bunk. Put dill in your diet. Really.

NUTRITIONAL INFORMATION

1 cup (65 g), sprigs

Calories:	4
Fat:	0 g
Carbohydrate:	1.89 g
Dietary fiber:	0 g
Sugars:	0 g
Protein:	0 g

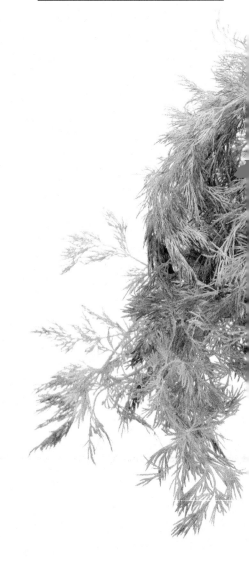

YOU NEED TO EAT THIS

BEAT BAD BREATH

This one may be too easy. Beyond just bad breath, some guys have bacteria in their mouth that causes halitosis. You can beat that by chewing dill. It won't just cover the smell; it will actually seek out the bacteria and kill the little buggers while you chew.

STOMACH PAIN RELIEF

If you've ever experienced a mild or severe stomach pain, you're well aware that your gut can stop you dead in your tracks no matter how healthy you are. Dill fights off diarrhea, relieves cramps, reduces acid reflux, and can ease just about any stomach pain, including excess gas or simply loss of appetite.

FIND CALM

Want more sleep? Want to reduce tension? Just want to calm yourself down? The essential oils found in dill are the answers to your stress-filled days, pal.

★ = serving of green food

DILL VEGETABLE DIP ★

½ cup (115 g) organic, whole sour cream

2 tablespoons (30 ml) lemon juice

1 teaspoon (1 g) of dried dill or 4 teaspoons (5 g) of fresh dill

Black pepper to taste

Combine all of the ingredients and serve as a dip for vegetables.

DILL SALMON BURGERS ★

1 can (6 ounces (170 g)) wild salmon

1 whole egg

¼ cup (40 g) red onion, chopped

1 lemon, juiced

1 tablespoon (4 g) chopped dill

3 tablespoons (33 g) Dijon mustard

Mix all of the ingredients in a bowl. Form into burgers. Bake these at 350°F (180°C or gas mark 4) for 15 minutes.

Easy Add-Ons to Your Diet

1. Use when cooking fish.
2. Use in salads, soups, and stir-fry dishes.
3. Chew for fresher breath.

STORAGE TIPS

• Store in the refrigerator either wrapped in a damp paper towel or with its stems placed in a container of water.

• Dill is fragile so it will only keep fresh for about two days.

FENNEL

If there's one thing about green foods, they're probably not going to entice your attention like a steak or a plate of nachos. Fennel is a prime example of this. While on the surface it looks like any old sprout out of your wife's vegetable garden, a closer look will show that the actual bulb of fennel is totally different. You don't have to love its look or taste to benefit from it though. Try it as a tea or simply in a stir fry and you'll be having better, longer sex and living long enough to enjoy it.

NUTRITIONAL INFORMATION

1 cup (100 g)

Calories:	27
Fat:	0.2 g
Carbohydrate:	6 g
Dietary fiber:	2.7 g
Sugar:	0 g
Protein:	1.1 g

YOU NEED TO EAT THIS

FIGHT CANCER

Fennel could be your ticket to beating colon cancer. It's also anticarcinogenic, which means it can be a huge resource for people undergoing radiation or chemotherapy treatments.

BETTER SEX

Known for years as a libido booster, fennel has been proven to increase sexual desires in both males and females. For men specifically, it can relieve bladder and prostate issues, prolong orgasms, and ultimately make men last longer.

STRENGTHEN YOUR STOMACH

Fennel can help in a myriad of stomach ailments including colic, heartburn, indigestion, spasms of the digestive tract, and painful gas, while also acting as an appetite suppressant. Fennel can also help gastric motility and aid in beating Irritable Bowel Syndrome (IBS).

STORAGE TIPS

• First, wash your fennel with cold water. Pat it dry and cut the stalks from the bulb.
• The outer layer may have a stringy consistency, so you can opt to peel it off with a vegetable peeler.

COOKING TIPS

• If the fennel is going to be used in dishes such as salads, or in dishes that require short cook times, slice the bulb thinly.
• If the fennel will be roasted or braised, chop the bulb in half to make wedges.
• The core can be removed if the cooking time is brief, but with longer cook times, the core will become soft.

★ = serving of green food

FENNEL, PEAR, AND GINGER JUICE ★ ★ ★

2 inches (5 cm) fresh ginger

½ bulb fennel

1 pear, cored

4 fresh mint leaves

Process all of the ingredients through a juicer. Serve cold.

DIGESTION SMOOTHIE ★ ★ ★

½ cup (120 ml) coconut milk or ½ cup (120 ml) water

1 cup (100 g) roughly chopped fennel bulb
   (approximately one small fennel bulb, cored)

1 small pear, cored

2 leaves of dinosaur kale (roughly chopped
   into 2 inch (5cm) pieces)

1 tablespoon (14 g) almond butter (add more to thicken)

Blend all of the ingredients on high, until smooth.

FENNEL MINT TEA ★ ★

10 to 12 mint leaves

4 cups (950 ml) water

Handful of fennel fronds (the feathery leaves) and seeds

Put the water in a tea kettle and heat until boiling.
Add the mint leaves and fennel fronds and seeds.
Let this steep for 20 minutes. Put mixture through
a sieve to remove herbs.

Easy Add-Ons to Your Diet

1. Shave fennel and add to salads for a delicious
   licorice flavor.
2. Caramelize onions and fennel and add to
   protein served at meals for a tasty combo.
3. Add to stir-fry dishes.
4. Chop fennel and add to soup for
   another flavor.
5. Chew fennel seeds after meals to help with
   digestion and soothe upset stomachs.

GREEN APPLE

We'll spare you the cliché about an apple a day and simply note that green apples are a staple of any healthy diet. We recommend you eat the skin so you can get the full benefit. Wash the skin before eating. If you slice them up and hate the browning that eventually develops, squirt some lemon juice on top and they're good as new.

NUTRITIONAL INFORMATION

1 medium, 3-inch (7.5-cm) diameter

Calories:	95
Fat:	0.31 g
Carbohydrate:	25 g
Dietary fiber:	4.4 g
Sugar:	19 g
Protein:	0.47 g

YOU NEED TO EAT THIS

WHITER TEETH

Chewing and biting an apple stimulates the production of saliva, which reduces bacteria in your mouth and, as a result, tooth decay. Apples, especially the dense green variety, act as a backup toothbrush and keep your teeth healthier and whiter.

MORE ENERGY

One of the quickest ways to boost your energy levels is by ingesting fructose. Before you reach for a soda, you've got to realize that the sugars you find in most processed foods and drinks is composed of high fructose corn syrup—essentially garbage sugar. Apples are packed with natural fructose—the real thing—so you'll get an energy spike from that as well as from the vitamin C and powerful antioxidants that you'll also be getting from your little green buddy.

STAY SHARP

Studies suggest that eating green apples can help combat Alzheimer's and Parkinson's diseases. Ultimately, they help slow down the aging process of the brain, which will keep your brain out of the fog and ready to go at a high level for years to come.

Easy Add-Ons to Your Diet

1. Add peanut or almond butter to slices for a great pre- or post-workout snack.
2. Slice very thin and add to salads for a flavor and vitamin boost.
3. Add to Greek yogurt or use slices of apple as a dipper.

GO ORGANIC

NON-ORGANIC APPLES ARE GREAT, BUT WHAT YOU CAN'T SEE ON THE SKIN OF YOUR FRESH FRUIT DOES LIMIT THE HEALTH BENEFITS. APPLES ARE IN THE TOP TWELVE FOODS WITH THE MOST PESTICIDE RESIDUES. ORGANICS WON'T HAVE THAT PROBLEM, AND THEY'LL HAVE 15 PERCENT MORE ANTIOXIDANTS FOR YOU TO BE HEALTHIER THAN EVER.

STORAGE TIPS

• Store ripe apples in your fridge's crisper to slow ripening and maintain crispness, but toss any bruised or moldy ones that might be sitting in there from last week's grocery run.

• Apples ripen much faster when stored at room temperature. Don't store them with leafy greens because the ethylene gas produced by apples as they mature can damage your greens. But this gas can speed the ripening process of pears and bananas—just throw an apple in a paper bag with these and they'll ripen quicker.

★ = serving of green food

GREEN APPLE AND GINGER SMOOTHIE ★ ★
1 green apple, cored and chunked
½ cup (15 g) frozen spinach
½ inch (1.3 cm) piece peeled fresh ginger, chopped
10 ounces (285 ml) water
Blend all of the ingredients on high, until smooth.

GREEN APPLE SALSA ★ ★ ★ ★
1 cup (125 g) green apple, chopped
⅔ cup (80 g) celery, diced
⅔ cup (45 g) cucumbers, diced
⅔ cup (110 g) red onion, diced
¼ cup (4 g) fresh cilantro, minced
¼ cup (60 ml) apple cider vinegar
2 tablespoons (30 ml) lemon juice
¼ teaspoon salt
Mix all of the ingredients together and serve with chips.

PB BITES ★
1 green apple; peanut butter; ground flaxseed
Cut the apple into slices. Spread peanut butter on the slices. Sprinkle with flaxseed.

GET YOUR PHYLL SMOOTHIE ★ ★ ★ ★ ★ ★ ★
If you've had a totally greenless day, plan on this smoothie at night to catch up and pack seven servings of green foods into one drink.
2 cups (60 g) spinach
1 green apple
1 kiwi
½ avocado
2 tablespoons (8 g) fresh parsley
1 tablespoon (15 g) spirulina powder
6 ounces (175 ml) water or coconut water

Blend all of the ingredients on high, until smooth.
NOTE: It can be tempting to go light on the greens and heavy on the fruit. You know you are making the smoothie correctly, and adding enough greens when the smoothie is actually bright green in color.

GREEN BEANS

Most of the time, the green beans on your table are drowning in butter or are a part of a mayonnaise-infused salad of some kind. Green beans, however, do not need dairy to be part of a great meal. In fact, green beans can be one of the most versatile foods you can include in a healthy diet. They're great as snacks, part of a salad, side dish, or even mixed into your main course.

NUTRITIONAL INFORMATION

1 cup (100 g)	
Calories:	34
Fat:	0 g
Carbohydrate:	8 g
Dietary fiber:	4 g
Sugars:	2 g
Protein:	2 g

YOU NEED TO EAT THIS

STRONGER BODY

You're only as strong as the weakest part of your body. For most guys, joints are a serious concern—especially after years of weight lifting and playing sports. Green beans can help strengthen your joints, bones, and connective tissue because they're a great source of silicon. Adding this to your diet will all but erase all your aches and pains and make you more fit in the process.

PRIMED MUSCLES

Green beans are packed with iron that helps oxygen flow through your lungs and around your bloodstream. This will ensure your brain and all your muscles are working at top condition. Green beans are also a protein source that is very low in calories. Snack on this and you'll be burning calories while fueling your muscle gains.

HEALTHIER LOOKING SKIN

Your wife applies collagen-laced cosmetics to her face. You don't. What you can do is eat green beans and make your skin look better from the inside out because by doing so, you'll be taking in some of nature's best collagen.

★ = serving of green food

HONEY CASHEW GREEN BEANS ★ ★

2 cups (200 g) fresh green beans, trimmed

2 tablespoons (18 g) coarsely chopped cashews

3 teaspoons (15 ml) coconut oil

1 tablespoon (20 g) raw honey

Place the green beans in a steamer basket. Place this in a saucepan over 1 inch (2.5 cm) of water and bring to a boil. Cover and steam until crisp tender. In a small skillet, sauté cashews in the coconut oil for about 2 minutes or until golden brown. Stir in the honey and heat through. Transfer the beans to a serving bowl and toss to coat. Serve immediately.

GREEN BEAN FRIES ★ ★

2 cups (200 g) green beans, trimmed

1 tablespoon (15 ml) coconut oil

Salt and pepper

Coat the green beans in coconut oil and season with salt and pepper. Bake on 400°F (200°C or gas mark 6) for 20 minutes, but turn at 15 minutes. They are done when there are brown spots and they are somewhat shriveled.

SPICY GREEN BEANS ★ ★ ★

2 cups (200 g) green beans, trimmed

Salt and pepper

3 tablespoons (45 ml) olive oil

2 cloves garlic, thinly sliced

¼ to ½ teaspoon crushed red pepper

Cook the green beans in boiled salted water until tender. Drain when finished. Wipe out the saucepan and heat the oil and garlic over medium heat for 2 minutes. Add the green beans, salt, and pepper, and toss to combine. Sprinkle with the crushed red pepper.

Easy Add-Ons to Your Diet

1. Eat raw as a snack between meals.
2. Sauté with onions and tomato and add to protein of choice.
3. Add to salads or use as a dipper.

STORAGE TIPS

• When preparing fresh green beans for storage, the pods should be placed unwashed in a plastic bag. If the beans are whole, they can be kept in the refrigerator for about seven days.

• When freezing and storing fresh green beans, it is recommended to first steam the beans for two to three minutes. Once the beans have been removed from heat and thoroughly cooled, place them in freezer bags and then store them in the freezer.

PREP TIP

• To prepare green beans for cooking, rinse the beans under running water. The ends should then either be cut off with a knife or snapped off. The healthiest method to cook green beans is by steaming them whole in a pot filled with 2 inches (5 cm) of boiling water for five minutes.

WHICH BEAN?

GREEN BEANS, LIKE MOST VEGETABLES, ARE BEST PURCHASED FRESH IF POSSIBLE. HOWEVER, FROZEN AND CANNED BEANS CAN STILL PROVIDE MANY BENEFICIAL NUTRIENTS. FRESH GREEN BEANS CAN RETAIN A HIGH NUTRIENT CONTENT AFTER FREEZING FOR THREE TO SIX MONTHS. GREEN BEANS THAT HAVE BEEN FROZEN AND THEN COOKED CAN RETAIN UP TO 90 PERCENT OF VITAMINS B6 AND B12, WHILE CANNED GREEN BEANS CAN LOSE ABOUT ⅓ OF THEIR PHENOLIC COMPOUNDS AND SMALL QUANTITIES OF B VITAMINS INCLUDING FOLIC ACID. IF PURCHASING FRESH GREEN BEANS, IT'S ADVANTAGEOUS TO BUY THEM FROM STORES THAT SELL THEM LOOSE TO PICK OUT THE BEST LOOKING BEANS. QUALITY GREEN BEANS ARE BRIGHT GREEN IN COLOR, AND ARE FIRM AND SMOOTH TO THE TOUCH WITHOUT ANY BROWN SPOTS OR DISCOLORATION.

GREEN GRAPES

Is there anything more regal than being fed green grapes? Well, we can't guarantee anyone will feed you grapes, but we do recommend you eat them as often as you can. They're packed with all the goodness you've grown to expect from the greens in this book. They're also one of the very best snacks for people who are on the go and want to lose weight or be pampered like an emperor—you know who you are.

NUTRITIONAL INFORMATION

1 cup (150 g)

Calories:	104
Fat:	0.2 g
Carbohydrate:	27 g
Dietary fiber:	1.4 g
Sugar:	23 g
Protein:	1.1 g

YOU NEED TO EAT THIS

FOR SUNSCREEN

Protect your skin from the inside by chowing down on some green grapes. These little guys will fend off the negative effects of UV radiation because of the powerful polyphenols they're packed with that prevent photocarcinogenesis on our skin.

BOUNCE BACK

Green grapes will replenish electrolytes that help with fluid balance and proper acidity of the blood. These electrolytes also help replenish the body after a strenuous workout or any physical activity. That means you'll bounce back faster and be ready to go sooner.

HYDRATE AND BOOST ENERGY

Grapes are 80 percent water so they act as a great hydrator when included in your diet. Because they're also low on the glycemic index, they'll release glucose into your system slower and thus boost your energy levels way longer than any sugar-packed energy drink or snack.

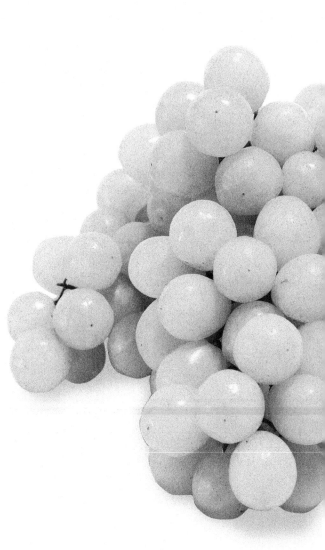

★ = serving of green food

PRE-WORKOUT SMOOTHIE ★ ★ ★
1 cup (150 g) seedless green grapes
1 banana
1 cup (30 g) spinach, raw
½ cup (120 ml) water, ice
Blend all of the ingredients on high, until smooth.

SAUTÉED GRAPES AND GOAT CHEESE ★ ★ ★
2 ounces (55 g) goat cheese, balled
1 cup (150 g) green grapes, sliced in half
½ tablespoon (2 g) oregano, fresh, chopped
½ tablespoon (1.2 g) thyme, fresh, chopped
Roll the goat cheese into small balls and place them on a plate. Sauté the grapes over medium heat on stove top in coconut oil until warm, about one minute. Pour the grapes onto the goat cheese balls. Add oregano and thyme and serve immediately.

THE "HJ" ★ ★ ★
BY KRISTINA SCIARRA, OWNER, HARVEST JUICERY
2 stalks celery
1 cup (30 g) spinach, raw
½ cup (75 g) grapes
Pinch of Portuguese salt cream or unrefined sea salt
Process all of the ingredients through a juicer.
Proportions should be: 2 parts spinach, 1 part celery, and 1 part grape

PISTACHIOS AND GRAPES ★ ★
Pistachios and green grapes

GREEN TRAIL MIX ★ ★
Green raisins and pistachios trail mix

Easy Add-Ons to Your Diet
1. Freeze and put in wine glasses to chill wine.
2. Roast with almonds and serve with crumbled goat cheese.
3. Add to oatmeal or broccoli salad.

BUYING AND STORAGE TIPS
• Grapes should be firm and snug to their stem. Grab the bunch and give it a shake. If lots of grapes fall, it's probably not the freshest. Look for a slight yellow tinge in color and avoid any that are browning.
• Make sure to refrigerate in a plastic bag and wash thoroughly before eating.

GREEN ONIONS

They may look like deformed grass cylinders, but green onions, also known as scallions, have a lot going for them beyond stinking less than the big white or red onions you're used to. They have 100 times more phytonutrients than their cousins and, since they have fewer layers to peel off and discard—and the outside layers have the most benefits—they're actually more nutritious for you. And they're easy to eat: Chop them and eat them. Or, if you're feeling fancy, steam them very lightly. Hard enough for you?

YOU NEED TO EAT THIS

BETTER VISION

Compared to white onions, green onions contain higher amounts of carotenoids, namely vitamin A, lutein, and zeaxanathin, which are especially important for eye health. Lutein and zeaxanathin work together to prevent cell damage and fight macular degeneration and can prevent corneal ulcers, as well as night blindness.

HEART HEALTH AND DEPRESSION KILLER

Green onions are packed with folate, which has been shown to reduce levels of homocysteine in men that is linked to a reduction in heart disease and risk of stroke. Low levels of folate are also common in men who are depressed, so adding in some green onions to your diet could prevent depression.

LOWER BLOOD PRESSURE

Onions are rich sources of phytonutrients, including quercetin, which is believed to have anti-inflammatory and antioxidant properties to block the creation of LDL cholesterol and to lower blood pressure.

NUTRITIONAL INFORMATION

1 tablespoon (10 g)

Calories:	1
Fat:	0 g
Carbohydrate:	0 g
Dietary fiber:	0 g
Sugar:	0 g
Protein:	0 g

★ = serving of green food

PEPPER AND ONION OMELETTE ★ ★
3 eggs
½ cup (75 g) green bell peppers, chopped
¼ cup (40 g) green onions, chopped
1 tablespoon (15 ml) refined coconut oil
4 ounces (115 g) chicken sausage (optional)
Whisk the eggs and pour them into a heated pan. Let eggs set. Cook on each side in the coconut oil, and then add the peppers and onions into the center. Fold it over the cooked egg into an omelet.

Easy Add-Ons to Your Diet

1. Include in nachos, soups, and stir-fry dishes.
2. Add to ground meat before cooking to add flavor.
3. Include in your scrambled eggs or simply top your protein in your main course.

STORAGE TIPS

• Green onions are easy to keep. Simply store them in a jar with some water on your counter or in your fridge.
• If the jar route isn't your style, wrap them in a paper towel and put them in your fridge's crisper.

GREEN PEAS

Here's something you may not know about green peas: They're actually legumes, not vegetables. Here's something you'll actually care about: Peas can be a fundamental building block in your quest to look your best, aiding in losing weight, building muscle, and helping you live a long, healthy life.

YOU NEED TO EAT THIS

PROTEIN PUNCH

One cup (145 g) of green peas contains 8 grams of protein, which is much higher than other greens, such as kale and spinach. You need protein to feed your muscles, and adding peas to your daily dose will yield results. Research has also found that pea protein could prolong the onset of kidney disease in people with high blood pressure.

MUSCLE UP

Peas are full of vitamins, such as vitamin C (one serving packs 96 percent or your daily recommended intake), vitamin A (one serving will stock you up with 22 percent of your daily dose), and lutein, which protects your cells from the type of damage that can occur after a workout. Helping your body overcome these stresses will ensure rapid gains.

FILL UP AND DROP WEIGHT

A great source of fiber with 7 grams per cup, peas will fill you up and keep you full. That means less snacking. Less snacking means less fat around your middle. Less fat around your middle means a longer life and more attention from your significant other.

NUTRITIONAL INFORMATION

1 cup (145 g)

Calories:	118
Protein:	8 g
Fat:	0.6 g
Carbohydrate:	21 g
Dietary fiber:	7 g
Sugar:	8 g

SNAP TO IT
WHEN PREPARING FRESH PEAS TO BE COOKED, THE BEST WAY TO REMOVE THE PEAS FROM THEIR PODS IS TO SNAP THE TOP AND PULL THE THREAD ON THE SIDES OF THE PODS.

★ = serving of green food

ROSEMARY GREEN PEA SALAD ★ ★ ★ ★

2 cups (260 g) frozen green peas, thawed

¾ cup (90 g) dried cranberries

4 teaspoons (2.8 g) chopped fresh rosemary

½ cup (120 ml) olive oil

¼ cup (60 ml) red wine vinegar

Salt and pepper to taste

After the peas are thawed, combine peas, cranberries, rosemary, olive oil, and red wine vinegar in bowl. Stir and coat the ingredients evenly in oil and vinegar. Add salt and pepper to taste.

GREEN POTATO CAKES ★ ★

1 cup (225 g) mashed potatoes

1 egg, lightly beaten

½ cup (15 g) spinach, chopped

¼ cup (32 g) green peas, lightly mashed

1 tablespoon (4 g) fresh parsley, chopped

2 tablespoons (30 ml) coconut oil

In a mixing bowl, stir together the mashed potatoes, egg, spinach, peas, and parsley. Form into balls about the size of golf balls, and flatten into cakes. Pan fry in the coconut oil, turning once, until golden-brown.

Easy Add-Ons to Your Diet ~~~~~~~

1. Warm with some sea salt and olive oil as a side dish or include in your other sides, such as potatoes or rice.
2. Include in stir-fry dishes or egg scrambles.
3. Sauté with other veggies to create a great side or add in protein of choice to make it into a main.

STORAGE TIPS

• The majority of green peas are either canned or frozen, fresh varieties are less common.

• Frozen green peas should ideally be consumed between six to twelve months after the packing date.

• Younger peas are starchier and more tender than mature peas.

GREEN PEPPER

Green peppers aren't spicy, aren't necessarily sweet, and are essentially young red peppers. That might not excite you, but eating these peppers will make you healthier. The green ones have been proven to have more phenolics than red ones. Something that'll keep you living longer.

NUTRITIONAL INFORMATION

½ cup (75 g), sliced

Calories:	9
Fat:	0 g
Carbohydrate:	2.13 g
Dietary fiber:	0.8 g
Sugar:	1.10 g
Protein:	0.40 g

YOU NEED TO EAT THIS

FOR SNACKING

Because of their near perfect nutritional profile, green peppers are a great snack that can boost your energy levels, fill you up without consuming a lot of calories, and aid in weight loss.

INSTANT BOOST

Vitamin C is an all-star. It boosts your immune system and helps your body run at its very best, no matter how you're treating it. When you're thinking about vitamin C, you're probably imagining an orange, but a green pepper has more than your daily recommended intake of the stuff, so slice it up and enjoy being healthy with what could possibly be considered the new orange juice!

CLEAR SKIN

Green peppers contain quercetin. You don't need to know how to spell it or pronounce it. All you need to know is that it'll make your skin look better.

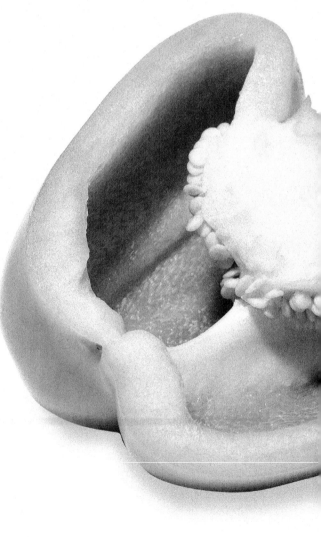

★ = serving of green food

BAKED GREEN PEPPERS ★

1 green pepper

Garlic salt

Pre-heat your oven to 400°F (200°C or gas mark 6). Cut the green pepper into strips and place them on a baking pan. Bake until slightly tender. Dip in hummus, salsa, guacamole, or dip of your choice.

OATMEAL FOR MEN ★ ★

1 cup (80 g) cooked oatmeal, gluten free

1 cup (150 g) green peppers, sautéed (add any greens)

2 teaspoons (10 ml) coconut oil

1 egg, served any style

Salt and pepper

Cook the plain oats with water. Add your choice of steamed or sautéed veggies to the oatmeal. Top with an egg for extra protein and season with salt and pepper.

GREEN PEPPERS AND HUMMUS ★

1 cup (150 g) green peppers or broccoli and hummus

OPTIONAL: Mix or blend chopped olives in the hummus.

EGG-STUFFED GREEN PEPPER ★

2 eggs

1 green pepper

2 ounces (55 g) diced, cooked bacon or other breakfast sausage

Cut off the top and hollow out a green pepper and fill it with two cracked whole eggs and cooked bacon or sausage. Sprinkle this with salt and pepper. Bake until the eggs are cooked through.

GRASS-FED STEAK FAJITAS

4 to 6 ounces (115 to 165 g) steak , grass fed

1 cup (150 g) green peppers, chopped

½ cup (80 g) onions, chopped

1 clove garlic, chopped

Cumin and chili powder to taste

Sear the grass-fed steak strips in a pan, and then finish cooking in the oven at 350°F (180°C or gas mark 4). Then, sauté the peppers and onions in the coconut oil. Add chopped garlic, cumin, and chili powder. Put the steak back into the pan with the cooked vegetables. Cook a few more minutes, then serve.
AND ONE: Serve with a side of guacamole.

Easy Add-Ons to Your Diet

1. Stuff with rice or quinoa, and ground protein for a great meal.
2. Include in salsa, guacamole, stir-fry dishes, or egg scrambles.
3. Sauté with other veggies to create a great side or add in protein of choice to make it into a main.

STORAGE TIPS

• Store fresh green peppers in a plastic bag in your vegetable crisper and they'll last about two weeks.
• If you're freezing, slice or chop peppers and spread them flat in an airtight container or heavy-duty freezer bags. Surprisingly, they'll be good for almost a year.

GREEN TEA

It would be easier to tell you what green tea doesn't do to improve your health. It won't grow back any severed limbs. That's about it. If you haven't heard how green tea can help you in literally hundreds of ways, you haven't been stepping out of your man cave enough. So let's forge new ground: Make some tea.

YOU NEED TO EAT THIS

FOR WEIGHT LOSS
Ever heard of catechin? Don't worry. Green tea is full of it, and it's been proven to help reduce body fat—especially around your belly. Want an even greater boost in your fat loss journey? Try matcha, a powder made from whole green tea leaves.

MENTAL CLARITY
Green tea contains theanine, which is a stimulant that supercharges your brain's neurotransmitters to increase your alpha brainwave activity. It makes you calm, while helping you concentrate. The effect can last for up to four hours.

BEAT BAD BREATH
Polyphenols fight bacteria in your mouth that cause bad breath. Guess what drink is full of these polyphenols? Green tea. Your co-workers and your lady will thank you.

NUTRITIONAL INFORMATION

8 ounces (235 ml), brewed

Calories:	2
Fat:	0 g
Carbohydrate:	1 g
Dietary fiber:	0 g
Sugar:	0 g
Protein:	0 g

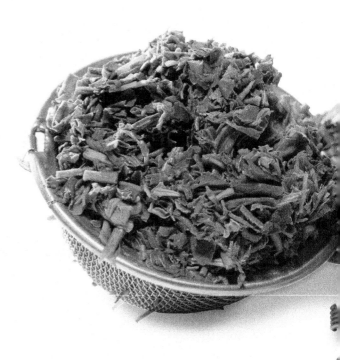

★ = serving of green food

6-HOUR ENERGY SMOOTHIE ★ ★ ★
1 medium Banana
2 tablespoons (28 g) almond butter
2 cups (60 g) spinach, fresh
8 to 10 ounces (235 to 285 ml) chilled green tea
Blend all of the ingredients on high, until smooth.

PRODUCTIVI-TEA ★ ★
8 ounces (235 ml) green tea
2 mint leaves
Make green tea and add 2 mint leaves. Steep for 3 to 4 minutes and remove tea bag and mint.

GREEN TEA SMOOTHIE ★ ★ ★ ★ ★ ★ ★
2 cups (60 g) spinach
1½ cups (355 ml) green tea, chilled
2 cups (300 g) frozen green grapes
2 teaspoons (10 g) raw honey
1 ripe avocado
Blend all of the ingredients together until smooth.

Easy Add-Ons to Your Diet
1. Replace your morning coffee with green tea.
2. Include it in your blended shakes.
3. Mix with mint and fruit for a fresh, nutrient-dense pick me up.

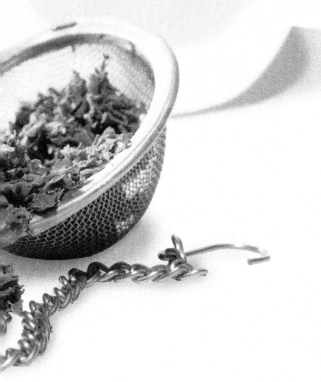

STORAGE AND PREP TIPS
• It is best to buy loose tea because it is higher in quality than those found in packaged bags, which are often laced with inferior quality leaves and branches. Store your tea in a dark cabinet or completely opaque container or resealable zipped bag.

• If you leave a green tea bag in hot water too long, it will have a strong bitter taste. Sometimes it only takes two to three minutes to be ready to drink. Loose tea needs even shorter time than a tea bag. If you want to serve your tea chilled or over ice, we recommend including some fresh fruit or some raw honey to sweeten your drink.

GUAVA

The last time you went to Mexico, you experienced a few things: Tequila only gives you a hangover if you stop drinking, buffet isn't such a great thing after your fourth day, and they've got some really incredible fruit. One of those fruits you loved so much was the guava. Flavor aside, take a look at the benefits listed here and you'll learn to love guava a lot more.

NUTRITIONAL INFORMATION

1 cup (140 g)

Calories:	112
Fat:	1.6 g
Carbohydrate:	24 g
Dietary fiber:	9 g
Sugars:	15 g
Protein:	4.2 g

YOU NEED TO EAT THIS

TO BEAT PROSTATE CANCER

More than just about any other food you'll find at the produce counter, guava is a lycopene superstar. Way more, in fact than watermelon or tomato. And lycopene is one antioxidant you can't skimp on—it specifically targets and fights prostate cancer.

AS A RESET

Consider guava as your body's reset button. Packed with vitamin A and C, flavonoids, and soluble dietary fiber, guava can rebuild just about any damage your body has undergone over the years. It'll boost your immunity against potential disease, build collagen to repair your skin, act as a serious laxative to improve your bowel health, and ultimately make you look and feel younger. It's also a prime source of copper, manganese, and magnesium, which will improve mental health, as well as blood vessel and nerve function.

BUYING AND STORAGE TIPS

• Your nose is your best tool when you're picking out guavas. The richer the scent, the better the fruit. If your nose isn't enough, look for tight skin that has a slight give to it under pressure from your palm.
• Make sure the skin has little to no spots.
• Green guavas (unripe) should be stored at room temperature, and ripe ones (yellowish-green) should be left in your fridge.

★ = serving of green food

GUAVA PAPAYA SMOOTHIE ★ ★

1 cup (140 g) ripe papaya

2 small guavas

1 sprig parsley

1 teaspoon (5 ml) lemon juice

½ teaspoon ginger

1 teaspoon (5 ml) Grade B maple syrup (optional)

3 to 4 ice cubes (optional)

Blend all of the ingredients until smooth.

Easy Add-Ons to Your Diet

1. Purée and mix with Greek yogurt to make your own dressing.
2. Juice guava with other tropical fruits to make a refreshing drink.
3. Dice and mix into your salsa, oatmeal, or cereal.

HONEYDEW MELON

Great as part of any fruit salad, honeydew has myriad health benefits, but beyond just being good for you, focus on how it's better for you. For one thing, it's sweet, and that makes it a great dessert that's better than any of the processed, sugar-filled deserts you usually go for. So get something sweet—slice off a piece of honeydew. It sure beats buying your snack from a vending machine.

NUTRITIONAL INFORMATION

1 cup (170 g)

Calories:	64
Fat:	0 g
Carbohydrate:	16 g
Dietary fiber:	1 g
Sugar:	14 g
Protein:	1 g

YOU NEED TO EAT THIS

LOWER BLOOD PRESSURE

Among the many benefits of eating this melon, you could also see an improvement if you've got high blood pressure. Why? Since honeydew is a good source of potassium, which helps regulate blood flow in your body, you'll be lowering your blood pressure without pills, just by stocking up on this sweet fruit.

BETTER SKIN

You may have heard that vitamin C can help you beat the flu, but did you know that it can help you look better? By boosting collagen levels in your system, honeydew consumption can help make your skin look younger and tighter.

★ = serving of green food

HONEYDEW MINT JUICE ★ ★ ★ ★

1 cup (170 g) honeydew melon, chopped

1 Granny Smith apple, cored

1 pear, cored

1 lemon

¼ cup (25 g) fresh mint

Process all of the ingredients through a juicer. Serve cold.

MINT MELON SALAD ★ ★ ★ ★

2 cups (340 g) honeydew

1 tablespoon (15 ml) fresh lime juice

⅔ cup (65 g) chopped fresh mint leaves

Cut the honeydew into 1-inch (2.5-cm) chunks. Drizzle the lime juice over the top and sprinkle mint. Mix and coat evenly.

Easy Add-Ons to Your Diet

1. Purée and mix with blueberries as a cold soup.
2. Dice and mix with arugula and mint as a tropical green salad.
3. Cut into cubes with other melons. Put cubes into a deep bowl that has a few shots of rum, vodka, or tequila. Let the fruits soak in the juice over night and serve as a snack.

STORAGE TIPS

• Store whole, ripe melons at room temperature or in the refrigerator for up to five days.

• Once cut, melon should be stored in a plastic bag (to prevent ethylene gas leakage) in the refrigerator for up to three days.

• If you're storing a cut melon, make sure it's placed in an airtight container so that it doesn't absorb odors from other foods.

JALAPEÑO

Guys like spice. And that's perfectly okay. But let's face it: The jalapeños you've been eating are probably not the best. They've been pickled or liberated from a can. What you really want to reach for are the fresh ones that actually have a red tint to them, so they haven't lost any of their vitamins and minerals. Great for so many meals and snacks, you'll hate yourself for not including these spicy buggers in your daily diet long ago.

NUTRITIONAL INFORMATION

1 pepper	
Calories:	4
Fat:	0 g
Carbohydrate:	1 g
Dietary fiber:	0.4 g
Sugar:	0.6 g
Protein:	0.1 g

YOU NEED TO EAT THIS

BURN FAT

Jalapeños are full of capsaicin, which is the chemical in peppers that makes your mouth feel like it's on fire. Beyond just burning your tongue, capsaicin has also been shown to increase your metabolism to help the weight loss process.

BETTER SEX

Eating jalapeños activate a receptor in our blood vessels that stimulates nitric oxide production, which leads to more and better erections.

WHITER TEETH

Noted as one of the best foods for oral care, jalapeños make your mouth water more than just about any other food you're eating. That extra saliva cleans your mouth and makes your pearly whites that much whiter.

STORAGE TIPS

- Store whole jalapeños in the fridge for about a week in a paper bag.
- If you want to freeze them, you can slice them up and put them in a sealed plastic bag and they'll last for a few months.

Easy Add-Ons to Your Diet

1. Add to nachos, salsa, guacamole, and any other dip.
2. Include in your egg scramble, sautéed veggies, or with your protein source for some added kick.
3. Add to salads and rice dishes or even inside sandwiches.

★ = serving of green food

JALAPEÑO COOLER JUICE ★ ★ ★ ★
½ pineapple
1 cup (16 g) cilantro
1 cucumber
½ lime
½ jalapeño

Process all of the ingredients through a juicer.

MEXICAN BREAKFAST PIZZA ★ ★
2 organic corn tostadas
1 avocado, mashed in a bowl
¼ cup (34 g) jalapeños, chopped
1 egg, fried in coconut oil

Spread the mashed avocado on the tostada. Mash in a bowl first, not on the tostada. Add the jalapeños. Top with fried egg in coconut oil (have a couple of these!).

SLOW COOKER CHICKEN TACOS ★
5 to 6 boneless chicken breasts
1 envelope taco seasoning
1 jar of salsa
½ cup (70 g) jalapeños

Place the chicken in the bottom of the slow cooker, pour salsa on top, and sprinkle with the taco seasoning and jalapeños. Cook on high for 4 to 6 hours or on low for 6 to 8 hours. When done, the chicken should shred easily when stirred with a fork. Serve with taco fixings!

KALE

Is there any one food that has been talked about more in the last few years than kale? Probably not. The truth is kale is everything all those fad diet types are claiming it to be. We're not suggesting you drop everything and be a tree-hugging, granola-eating hippie about it. Just make sure you get some before they eat it all up and you'll be glad you did—better sex, more muscle, and lower cholesterol are sure to follow.

NUTRITIONAL INFORMATION

1 cup (67 g), chopped

Calories:	33
Fat:	0.6 g
Carbohydrate:	6 g
Dietary fiber:	1 g
Sugar:	0 g
Protein:	2 g

YOU NEED TO EAT THIS

MORE MUSCLE

The chlorophyll found in kale helps increase red blood cell production and promotes tissue growth and repair. That means more muscle gains as your body repairs everything and grows in the process. It also helps limit your fatigue so you're ready to get back to it a lot sooner.

LOWER CHOLESTEROL

Including kale in your diet can lower your cholesterol—especially if it's already high and you're a man. Men who drank about a half a cup (120 ml) of kale juice each day for ninety days saw dramatic results, including lowered LDL and increased HDL and HDL to LDL ratios.

BEATING E.D.

Kale is such a powerful superfood that it can even help you in the sack. Research has shown that men have experienced increased blood flow and fewer problems with erectile dysfunction when they consume a diet that includes kale. They've also seen improved stamina and energy levels.

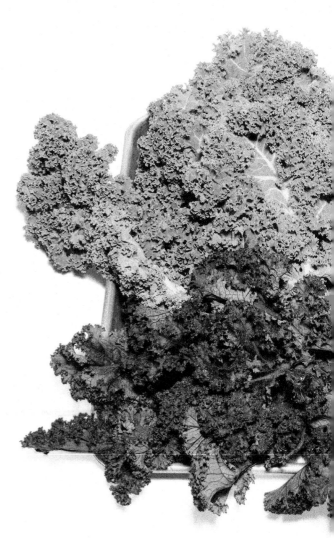

★ = serving of green food

DETOX JUICE ★ ★ ★ ★ ★
2 cups (134 g) kale
2 cups (142 g) broccoli
4 medium carrots
1 medium apple
Process all of the ingredients through a juicer. Serve cold.

KALE AND GREEN APPLE SMOOTHIE ★ ★ ★
4 kale leaves (stems removed)
2 cored apples (unpeeled)
1 cup (235 ml) almond milk
1 tablespoon (20 g) raw honey
Blend all of the ingredients on high, until smooth.

KALE CHIPS ★ ★
1 bunch kale
1 tablespoon (15 ml) olive oil
1 teaspoon (6 g) seasoning salt
Preheat oven to 350°F (180°C or gas mark 4). Line a cookie sheet with parchment paper. With a knife or kitchen shears, carefully remove the leaves from the thick stems and tear into bite size pieces. Wash and thoroughly dry kale with a salad spinner. Drizzle kale with olive oil and sprinkle with seasoning salt. Bake until the edges brown (approximately 10 to 15 minutes).

GREEN EGGS ★
2 eggs
2 large kale leaves (do not trim or remove stems)
Pinch Celtic Sea Salt
2 teaspoons (10 ml) coconut oil
Place the eggs, kale leaves, and salt in a blender. Blend on high until smooth. Cook the eggs using the coconut oil in frying pan and scramble.

Easy Add-Ons to Your Diet

1. Chop up and include in raw ground meats before cooking.
2. Include in your egg scramble, sautéed veggies, or with your protein source for some added kick.
3. Replace iceberg lettuce with kale and a mix of arugula and beet greens for a super-powered salad.
4. Make your own spin on guacamole by including kale in your mix.
5. Include in your smoothies and juices.

BUYING AND STORAGE TIPS
• Make sure you buy organic kale. The regular stuff has mostly likely been packed with pesticides.
• Pass on any leaves that are wilting, yellowing, or showing any brown color.
• Store kale in a sealed bag in your fridge for up to five days.
• Don't wash it until you're ready to eat it, as the washing process will promote wilting.

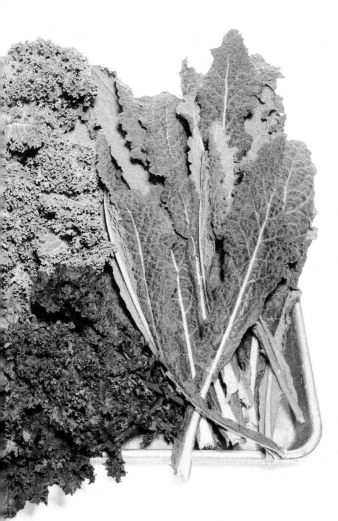

KIWI

The most unassuming fruit you'll ever see. That's what we're dubbing the kiwi. From the outside, it could pass for a rock or a rather hum drum, dry, and starchy vegetable. One slice past the fuzzy skin and you're welcomed with something extremely exotic and powerful.

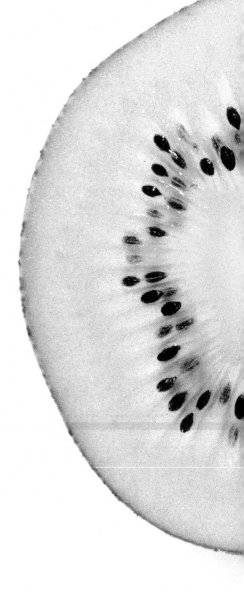

NUTRITIONAL INFORMATION

1 medium fruit (2 inches (5 cm))	
Calories:	42
Fat:	0.4 g
Carbohydrate:	10 g
Dietary fiber:	2 g
Sugar:	6 g
Protein:	0.8 g

YOU NEED TO EAT THIS

BETTER SEX
Whether you're impotent, too quick, not hard enough, or just not the man you used to be, kiwi can help you in the sack. Because these little green fruits are a good source of arginine, they act as a vasodilator, which will bring back your mojo and quite possibly give you better orgasms as well.

BE HAPPY
Recent research found that kiwi consumption could actually improve your mood. In fact, it can even combat depression. Subjects who ate just one helping of kiwi each day reported a one-third reduction in their depression symptoms. Those who ate more saw even greater results.

POST WORKOUT
Because kiwi is low in fructose, it makes for a great post-workout snack. Furthermore, research has shown that the vitamin C in kiwi performs better than that from oranges or grapefruits in repairing your body after intense physical activity.

BUYING AND STORAGE TIPS
• Most kiwi you find in the grocery store is under ripe. If you want to ripen them quickly, leave them out in room temperature for a couple of days.
• Stored in the fridge, you should expect your kiwi to last about a week.

★ = serving of green food

POST-WORKOUT SMOOTHIE ★ ★

1 cup (235 ml) tart cherry juice

2 medium kiwis

1 tablespoon (20 g) maple syrup

1 to 2 scoops protein powder—undenatured whey, grass-fed cow

Ice as needed

Unrefined seal salt (add pinch for trace minerals) and seaweed dulse flakes (optional)

Blend all of the ingredients on high, until smooth.

KIWI PURÉE ★

Using a food processor or blender, blend a peeled kiwi to make a simple fruit purée to top on Bancakes, pancakes, waffles, or French toast.

EGG "BANCAKES" WITH PURÉED KIWI ★ ★

2 eggs

1 mashed ripe banana

2 teaspoons (10 ml) coconut oil

2 medium kiwis

Cinnamon

Mash the eggs and ripe banana in a bowl (or blend with a food processor). Pour the batter into a pan and pan-fry in coconut oil. Sprinkle with cinnamon. Top with puréed kiwi.

IMMUNITY BOOST ★ ★ ★ ★

½ large avocado

2 kiwi, peeled

2 tablespoons (30 ml) lime juice

2 tablespoons to ¼ cup (30 to 60 ml) almond or coconut milk

1 tablespoon (20 g) raw honey

2 to 3 ice cubes

Place the liquid in the blender first, then the fruit and ice. Cover. Start on low speed, increasing to high speed. Blend it up until creamy and smooth.

Easy Add-Ons to Your Diet

1. Chop up and include in fruit salad.
2. Slice and include in morning dishes such as pancakes and waffles.
3. Purée and mix with Greek yogurt for a great post-workout snack that will help repair and build muscle.

LEEKS

Regarded as one of the oldest vegetables on the planet, leeks are related to onions and garlic, but lack the overpowering flavor and scent. What they don't lack, however, is nutritional value or culinary versatility. The bottom line: Eating leeks will make you healthier with each meal, specifically with relation to some of the most common health hazards for men. And it will add some punch to just about everything you eat.

NUTRITIONAL INFORMATION

1 cup (104 g)

Calories:	54
Fat:	0.3 g
Carbohydrate:	13 g
Dietary fiber:	1.6 g
Sugar:	3.5 g
Protein:	1.3 g

YOU NEED TO EAT THIS

PROSTATE PROTECTOR
The American Cancer Institute estimates nearly 30,000 men will die from prostate cancer in the United States in 2014. One of your best bets to avoid getting prostate cancer is to consume allium veggies like leeks. Allium vegetables are a family of vegetables that contain beneficial sulfer compounds that contribute to their aroma but also provide anti-cancer benefits. If you already have it, the good news is that some research indicates that it may still be helpful. Stock up!

DON'T SWEAT CHOLESTEROL
Bad cholesterol is called LDL. Good cholesterol is called HDL. If you don't want to ever have to worry about what they're called, make sure your diet is full of leeks as they lower the bad, raise the good, and even stabilize your blood sugar.

BEAT STRESS
Kaempferol might just be your biggest ally against hypertension and, you guessed it, leeks are full of the stuff. Basically, they protect your blood vessels and increase the production of nitric oxide, which relaxes your blood vessels and ultimately nips anxiety and hypertension in the bud.

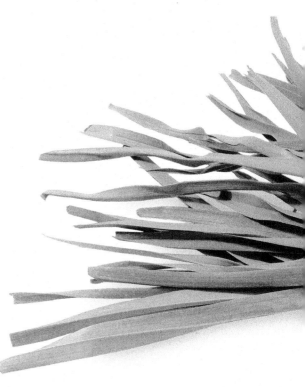

BUYING TIPS
• The tops of the leeks should be crisp and firm, with a dark green color. If they've begun to brown or dry out, leave them behind.
• The bottom of the leek should be a white bulb with roots sticking out. If it's cut or dry, it isn't fresh.

★ = serving of green food

SAUTÉED LEEKS ★

2 leeks, white and light-green parts only, halved length-
wise, and cut crosswise into 1-inch (2.5-cm) pieces

1 tablespoon (20 g) raw honey

1 teaspoon (5 ml) sherry or red wine vinegar

After cutting the leeks, place them in a heated skillet
with a little coconut oil over medium heat. Cook until
leeks are tender, about 8 minutes. Remove from heat.
Pour the honey and vinegar over and toss in salt and
pepper to taste.

KIWI LEEK APPLE SALAD ★ ★ ★ ★

1 leek, thinly sliced

¼ teaspoon garlic

Salt

2 kiwis peeled and diced

3 tablespoons (45 ml) flax oil

1 apple, thinly sliced

3 tablespoons (45 ml) extra-virgin olive oil

¼ teaspoon sea salt

Place all of the ingredients in a bowl and massage
together for 1 to 2 minutes. Let this sit for at least 1 hour
before serving.

Easy Add-Ons to Your Diet

1. Chop up and top your nachos, soup, and salads.
2. Slice and include in salsa, guacamole, and pasta sauces.
3. Sauté with mixed veggies and use as a side dish or as a base for a main.

LIME

Admit it: The last time you saw a lime may have been sticking out of a Corona bottle or on the rim of a rum and coke. We're not judging. We're just saying pass on the drinks, but keep the lime.

YOU NEED TO EAT THIS

CANCER KILLER

Limes are packed with flavonoids called flavonol glycosides that have been proven to prevent cell division in certain cancers. They also have limonoids, which early research shows to have a very positive impact on beating various forms of cancer, including skin, mouth, lung, and colon.

BEAT HEARTBURN

One thing guys know is heartburn. Ancient cultures had the solution long before you overindulged: lime juice. A couple teaspoons of lime juice added to hot water can make all that pain fade away—just be sure to make smarter food choices the next time.

DIGESTION

You know you're in for a good meal when your mouth is watering. You're also helping your body digest that meal when your mouth is watering. Saliva production is at its peak when you're about to scarf down your favorite meal or when you're having some tart lime juice. And, lime juice kicks up the preliminary digestion process.

NUTRITIONAL INFORMATION

1 fruit, 2 inches (5 cm) diameter

Calories:	20
Fat:	0 g
Carbohydrate:	7 g
Dietary fiber:	2 g
Sugar:	1 g
Protein:	0 g

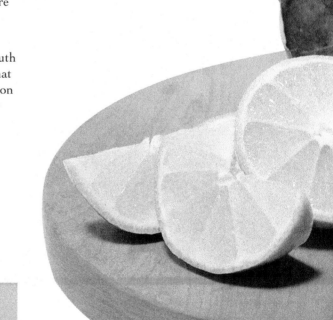

CORRECT YOUR SLICE
WHEN SLICING YOUR LIME, CUT IT IN HALF, NOT THROUGH THE STEM LIKE YOU NORMALLY WOULD WITH OTHER FRUITS.

★ = serving of green food

CHILI LIME PUMPKIN SEEDS ★ ★

1½ cups pumpkin seeds, raw

¼ teaspoon cayenne

¼ teaspoon black pepper

1 teaspoon (6 g) salt

3 tablespoons (45 ml) freshly squeezed lime juice

Mix the lime juice, pepper, cayenne, and salt and stir until dissolved. Heat a large skillet over medium heat. Add the pumpkin seeds and toss frequently until the seeds begin to turn light golden and expand. Add the liquid mixture and stir to coat all of the seeds. Let cool and serve at room temperature.

SUPER-GREEN SALAD ★ ★ ★ ★ ★

1 large avocado, sliced

4 scallions, sliced

Juice of ½ a lime

½ cup (60 g) cucumber cut into chunks

2 cups (60 g) fresh baby spinach leaves

Drizzle the avocado slices with the lime juice and set aside. Add the spinach, scallions, cucumbers, and avocado slice. Add a salad dressing, and toss.

Easy Add-Ons to Your Diet ~~~~~~

1. Squeeze liquid into water, add mint leaves and ice for a refreshing, detoxifying drink.
2. Mix juice with Greek yogurt and oregano to make a great dip or dressing.
3. Bake protein sources with slices of lime so the flavor is absorbed.
4. Add slices of lime, green apple, and oranges with some mint leaves to red or white wine and seltzer to make sangria.
5. Drizzle over grilled meats as you're cooking and after prepared.

STORAGE TIPS

• Limes can be kept out at room temperature where they will stay fresh for up to one week, if kept out of sunlight.

• Limes can be stored in the refrigerator crisper, wrapped in a loosely sealed plastic bag for ten to fourteen days. Although they can be kept longer than that, if left for another several weeks, they will begin to lose their characteristic flavor.

MINT

We know this may be a hard sell. We're telling you that leaves can positively affect your health. You're a man, and you don't want anything close to your mouth that's going to get you compared to a rabbit or bird. We understand. But, mint leaves aren't that easy to dismiss. You can find them in some of the best drinks at your local pub. You can also chow down on some of the best burgers and find that mint is what made them stand out so much. So, if you can get past the urge to ridicule this little leaf, you'll find some serious benefits that nearly nothing else can offer with so little work on your part, aside from chewing or chopping. You can do that, can't you?

NUTRITIONAL INFORMATION

2 tablespoons (12 g), fresh

Calories:	2
Fat:	0 g
Carbohydrate:	0.5 g
Dietary fiber:	0.3 g
Sugar:	0 g
Protein:	0.1 g

YOU NEED TO EAT THIS

MEMORY LOSS AND MENTAL CLARITY

Did you ever think that the simple act of chewing could improve the way your brain functions? Well, if you're chewing mint leaves or gum with mint extract as one its main ingredients, you'll be thinking clearer in no time. The simple act of ingesting mint in this manner has been proven to enhance your memory, make you more alert, and improve cognitive function.

FAT LOSS

Mint has long been known to be a stimulant, but recent studies indicate that it can also trigger fat loss and limit consumption. By triggering digestive enzymes in your mouth, mint can have a positive impact on your body's transformation of fat through the process of digestion. Bonus: It'll turn that fat into energy instead of letting it sit and be stored around your gut.

KILL STINK BREATH

We already talked about chewing mint (or mint-flavored gum), but we've got another positive coming from it: improved breath and oral hygiene. It's so good for you that your mouth, teeth, gums, throat, and breath will all see a marked improvement in no time.

CHOP THIS
THE EASIEST METHOD OF CHOPPING MINT IS TO ROLL THE LEAVES UP AND SLICE WITH A KNIFE.

STORAGE TIPS

• The most effective way to store mint in the refrigerator is to rinse the leaves off thoroughly, pat dry in paper towels, and place the wrapped bunch in airtight plastic bag. It'll keep for about a week.

★ = serving of green food

MINT MOJO JUICE ★ ★ ★ ★

1 cucumber

1 large pear

½ lime

¾ cup (12 g) fresh mint leaves

Process all of the ingredients through a juicer. Serve cold.

LIME AND MINT WATER ★ ★

Slice a lime and add it to water along with some whole mint leaves.

MINT TEA ★

Brew mint tea, and enjoy hot or cold.

LEMON MINT DRESSING ★ ★ ★

⅓ cup (160 ml) olive oil

2 tablespoons (30 ml) lemon juice

2½ tablespoons (15 g) chopped fresh mint leaves

½ clove garlic (optional)

Stir the olive oil, lemon juice, and chopped mint leaves together until well blended. Let dressing marinate for 2 hours before serving for best results.

Easy Add-Ons to Your Diet

1. Chop and add to ground meats before cooking.
2. Add chopped mint to salsa, pico de gallo, guacamole, or any salad or dressing.
3. Use as a garnish on virtually any dish, especially those with sauces.
4. Mix with Greek yogurt to make a dressing or dip.

OLIVE OIL

You probably pay more attention to the oil you're putting in your car than the oil on your plate. The truth is, there's even less to know about the oil on your plate than the one you're putting in your ride. All you need to know is that olive oil is a healthy fat and it can help you beat high cholesterol, improve your mood, and even make you more of a man. Bonus: You won't need to search for high performance fuel like you do for your new car. Get some now.

NUTRITIONAL INFORMATION

1 tablespoon (15 ml)

Calories:	120
Fat:	14 g
Carbohydrate:	0 g
Dietary fiber:	0 g
Sugar:	0 g
Protein:	0 g

YOU NEED TO EAT THIS

PAIN RELIEF

Extra-virgin olive oil is as effective for reducing inflammation as over the counter anti-inflammatory medicines. This powerful pain relief comes from oleocanthal, which is a special polyphenol in olive oil that can leave you feeling better in record time.

TESTOSTERONE BOOSTER

Been hearing a lot about low testosterone on TV lately? Maybe you've even been tempted to ask your doctor to check your levels out? Recent research indicates that men between the ages of 23 and 40 who consume olive oil regularly can increase their testosterone levels naturally by more than 15 percent. If you don't know what testosterone can help you with, then you don't know your body because it is the single most vital and unique element that makes you a man—and, ahem, what makes you most manly as well.

GET HAPPY

Getting happy could be as simple as getting a little greasy. Recent research discovered that people who consumed natural healthy fats such as olive oil reduced their risk of depression by nearly half compared to those that ate a diet with trans fats.

AVOID HIGH HEAT

PLEASE NOTE: OLIVE OIL ISN'T FOR COOKING AT HIGH TEMPERATURES. LIQUID OILS ARE UNSTABLE AT HIGH HEAT AND WILL CREATE FREE RADICALS (THE THINGS THAT AGE YOU FASTER). IT'LL ALMOST DEFINITELY START TO SMOKE BEFORE YOU'RE DONE COOKING. INSTEAD, USE OLIVE OIL FOR DRESSING, NON-COOKED DISHES, MIXES AND SALADS, OR DRIZZLE ON VEGETABLES AFTER STEAMING THEM.

★ = serving of green food

OLIVE OIL VINAIGRETTE ★
¼ cup (60 ml) balsamic vinegar

1 tablespoon (10 g) chopped garlic

¾ cup (175 ml) olive oil

½ teaspoon salt

½ teaspoon pepper

Place all of the ingredients in a screw-top jar and shake to combine. Serve with chicken and spinach salad.

KALE SUPER SALAD ★ ★ ★
3 cups (140 g) kale

1 cup (145 g) blueberries

½ medium avocado

4 to 6 ounces (115 to 165 g) chicken, salmon, or steak

2 tablespoons (30 ml) extra-virgin olive oil

2 tablespoons (30 ml) balsamic vinegar

1 teaspoon (5 g) raw honey

Combine the oil, vinegar, and honey first. Blend well. Drizzle on top of salad.

ROSEMARY BEETS IN OLIVE OIL ★ ★
Beets marinated in chopped rosemary and olive oil

SARDINES ★
Sardines packed in olive oil

BUYING AND STORAGE TIPS
• When buying olive oil, look for the dark bottles marked extra virgin.

• For the most health benefits, use it all up within the first few months. If it's been sitting around, it's time to get a new bottle.

• Store your oil in a dark area away from light and heat.

Easy Add-Ons to Your Diet
1. Drizzle on a plate with balsamic vinaigrette along with some oregano and use as a dip for fresh crusty bread.
2. Add to salads, pesto, or pasta dishes.
3. Use as a marinade with some wine for your protein.

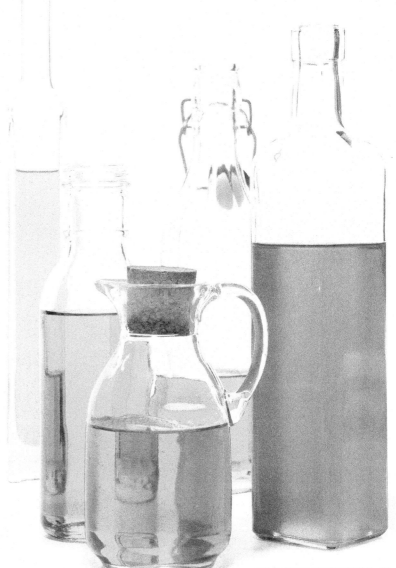

OLIVES

Olives are older than the city you're living in. Sound strange? Well, short of wine, there's little in this book or on any menu that could be considered as biblical or as historical as olives. Why should you care about that? Because they taste great and make you an even healthier big man. So make sure you've got some in your diet—and we mean more than what is in your martini.

NUTRITIONAL INFORMATION

1 ounce (28 g)

Calories:	41
Fat:	4 g
Carbohydrate:	1 g
Dietary fiber:	1 g
Sugars:	0 g
Protein:	0 g

YOU NEED TO EAT THIS

HEALTHY GUT

Eating a healthy diet that includes monounsaturated fats and getting your daily dose of vitamin E has been linked to a lesser risk of colon cancer. Olives offer up both and have been proven to beat ulcers and gastritis by activating the secretion of bile and pancreatic hormones better than anything your doctor can prescribe.

BETTER SKIN

Olives are great hydrators that do more than just infuse your body with water. They also protect your skin. If you're eating olives or applying an extract to your face, the high levels of vitamin E protect you from ultraviolet radiation. That means decreased risk of skin cancer and younger looking skin.

LOWER BLOOD PRESSURE

Olives can change the way your cells work and beat high blood pressure in the process. The oleic acid in these little green guys is absorbed by your body, gets into the cells, and starts making cell membrane level changes that help your blood pressure dip naturally. Science can be confusing, but it can also save your life.

STORAGE AND PREP TIPS

• Olives purchased in glass jars can be stored directly in the refrigerator after opening and will last one to two months.
• Canned olives that are purchased and not immediately consumed after opening can be stored in a sealed container in the refrigerator and can last one to two weeks.
• They come in a variety of liquids such as brine, acid, or water base, which should be transferred with the olives into the sealed container to store in the refrigerator.

PIT TIP
OLIVES CAN EASILY BE PITTED BY PRESSING DOWN ON THEM WITH THE FLAT SIDE OF A LARGE KNIFE.

★ = serving of green food

OLIVE SALSA ★ ★

1 cup (100 g) black olives, drained

1 cup (100 g) green olives, drained

2 cups (520 g) salsa

In a food processor, mince olives into small pieces. Mix with the salsa.

OLIVE TAPENADE ★ ★

1 cup (100 g) green olives, pitted and drained

1 tablespoon (8.6 g) drained capers

1 large garlic clove, minced

1 teaspoon (5 ml) fresh lemon juice

¼ cup (60 ml) olive oil

Combine all of the ingredients in a food processor, adding lemon and olive oil toward the end of blending.

MARINATED GREEN OLIVES IN OLIVE OIL ★ ★

Green olives marinated in olive oil.

CHIPS AND OLIVE SALSA ★

Tortilla, sweet potato, or sprouted grain chips with olive salsa

STUFFED OLIVES ★

Olives stuffed with tomatoes or roasted garlic

Easy Add-Ons to Your Diet

1. You can use crushed olives in hummus, bruschetta, or in a savory olive tapenade.
2. Add to stir frys, salads, and pasta dishes.
3. Use as an easy on-the-go snack.

OREGANO

The simple oregano leaf can build up your bones, help fight cancer, prevent blood clots, lower cholesterol, decrease fever, and make you look better. No wonder ancient Greeks referred to it as mountain joy and a symbol of happiness.

YOU NEED TO EAT THIS

ERASE PIMPLES
Your days of big zits manifesting on your face the night before prom may be over, but the occasional breakout can still be a pain in the butt. Topically applying oregano or oregano-based creams to your skin can calm even the most angry pizza face complexions. It'll even work wonders on dandruff.

BEAT THE BURN
If you've ever experienced a urinary tract infection, you know just how serious it can be. Beat those burning sensations from south of the belt line with a diet packed with oregano. Some folks opt for a tea-based drink in these cases, but the consumption of the leaf alone will help.

BACTERIA BUSTER
As an active guy, you're coming into contact with some nasty bacteria at the gym, on the court, and even in your own gym bag. Making sure you've got oregano in your diet can actually help beat all of them because of its antibacterial qualities.

NUTRITIONAL INFORMATION

1 tablespoon (4 g)

Calories:	9
Fat:	0 g
Carbohydrate:	2 g
Dietary fiber:	1 g
Sugar:	0 g
Protein:	0 g

★ = serving of green food

OREGANO WHITE BEAN SALAD ★ ★

1 can (15.5 ounces (440 g)) cannellini beans, rinsed and drained

1 large clove garlic, finely chopped

3 tablespoons (45 ml) extra-virgin olive oil

2 tablespoons (8 g) fresh chopped oregano or 1 tablespoon (3 g) dried

Salt and pepper to taste

Combine all of the ingredients in a bowl and serve.

FIVE-MINUTE ITALIAN DRESSING ★ ★ ★

½ cup (120 ml) olive oil

2 tablespoons (30 ml) lemon juice

1 clove garlic, minced

1 teaspoon (5 g) onion powder

1 teaspoon (5 g) raw honey

1 teaspoon (5 g) dried oregano

¼ teaspoon. dried basil

½ teaspoon sea salt

Combine all of the ingredients in a small container, cover, and shake well. Note that this dressing gets even stronger the longer it sits before use.

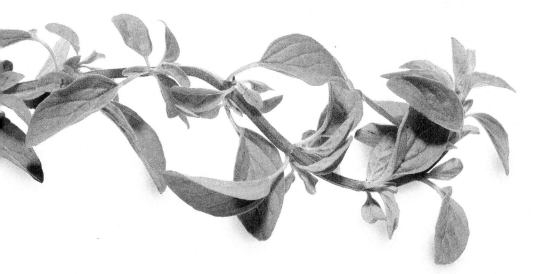

Easy Add-Ons to Your Diet

1. Add fresh leaves to a pizza instead of just dried. You can also add basil in this fashion.
2. Sauté with onions and mushrooms to make a great side or base for your main dishes.
3. Sprinkle into egg dishes, salsas, tomato sauces, and pasta dishes, as well as over salads and garlic bread.

BUYING AND STORAGE TIPS

• Fresh oregano is always a better option than dried. Avoid yellowing leaves with brown spots and make sure the stems are firm.

• Wrap oregano in a wet paper towel and store in your fridge.

• You can also freeze it in an airtight container.

• If you do opt for dried oregano, keep it in a sealed airtight container in a cupboard.

PARSLEY

You have to wonder about the first chef who used parsley as a garnish. Was he getting too cute with his plating, or was he secretly hoping to stifle the use of parsley as anything but a visual aid? Admit it: You've flicked it off your steak and went about eating without giving it a second thought. But it could help you in nearly every possible way that matters most to you as a man: virility, muscle growth, fat loss, cancer prevention, pain relief, staving off infection, and even making your breath smell great. Don't let that first chef's hate on parsley dictate how you should eat—and live!

NUTRITIONAL INFORMATION

1 tablespoon (4 g)

Calories:	1
Fat:	0 g
Carbohydrate:	0.2 g
Dietary fiber:	0.1 g
Sugar:	0 g
Protein:	0.1 g

YOU NEED TO EAT THIS

CIGARETTE NULLIFIER

If you're a smoker or someone who is subject to a lot of second-hand smoke, you'll want to make sure you've got some parsley in your diet. Parsley is what's called a chemoprotective herb that can help stop carcinogens from destroying your body. It is especially powerful in blocking the harmful effects of charcoal and cigarette smoke.

WEIGHT LOSS

Drop water weight with ease with the help of this diuretic. Besides just water weight, however, including parsley in your diet will positively impact your attempts to lose fat long term.

MUSCLE BUILDER

With three times as much vitamin C as oranges and twice as much iron as spinach, parsley is clearly something you need in your arsenal when you're trying to build muscle. Some research also indicates that this little herb may trigger the production of growth hormone, another vital element to getting bigger.

CLEAN GREENS
BEFORE EATING, MAKE SURE TO WASH AWAY ANY DIRT BY SWISHING IT AROUND IN A BOWL OF WATER.

BUYING AND STORAGE TIPS

Fresh parsley is easy to spot: bright green, firm stems, no yellowing or spots of any kind. Flat leaves are spicier than the more mild curly leaves. Store your parsley in a damp paper towel in your fridge.

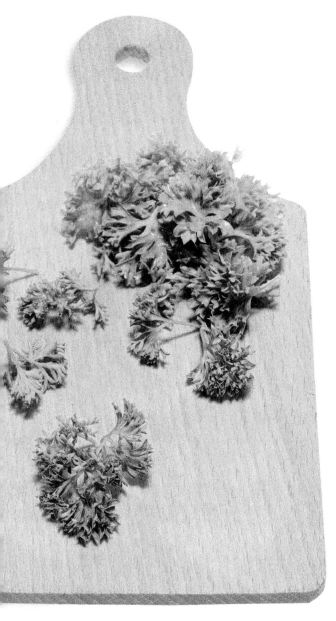

★ = serving of green food

DETOX SMOOTHIE ★ ★ ★
2 organic kale leaves
2 leaves fresh parsley
½ cucumber
1 cup (255 g) frozen strawberries
1 teaspoon (2 g) fresh ginger (peeled)
Blend all of the ingredients until smooth.

LEMON PARSLEY SAUCE ★ ★
2 lemons, juiced
5 tablespoons (75 ml) olive oil
3 tablespoons (12 g) parsley, finely chopped
Whisk all of the ingredients together. Serve on top
of fish or salad.

PHYLL UP JUICE ★ ★ ★ ★ ★ ★ ★
If you've had a totally greenless day, plan on this
smoothie at night to catch up and pack seven servings
of green foods into one drink.
2 celery stalks
1 broccoli trunk
1 green apple
1 bunch of parsley
½ cucumber
3 large romaine lettuce leaves
3 large kale leaves
Put all of the ingredients in your juicer.
Drink fresh and enjoy!

Easy Add-Ons to Your Diet

1. Add chopped parsley, garlic, lime zest, and
   olive oil together to create a great rub and
   marinade for chicken or steak.
2. Include in your pre-workout juices or
   smoothies for a spike of vitamins that are
   essential for gains.
3. Sprinkle over egg scrambles, fish and other
   protein dishes, salsas, pesto, hummus, tomato
   sauces, and pasta dishes.

PEAR

Pears have not been treated well by popular culture. Apples are lauded for their shape and are even considered naughty as a result of their cameo in the Bible. Pears, however, aren't sexy in the eye of the shared social consciousness. Packed with antioxidants, vital nutrients, and offering a light sweet flavor that no other fruit can compare with, pears should be in your top five fruits to reach for as often as you can.

NUTRITIONAL INFORMATION

1 medium pear	
Calories:	102
Fat:	0.2 g
Carbohydrate:	27 g
Dietary fiber:	6 g
Sugar:	7 g
Protein:	0.6 g

YOU NEED TO EAT THIS

CANCER FIGHTER

Pear skin is usually discarded, but eating it can actually help you beat colon cancer. The stone cells in pear skin can help reduce polyps, or growths, in your colon, which can reduce your risk of getting cancer.

HEALTHY HAIR

Of all the vital nutrients found in pears, you can't discount the importance of the copper it contains. Full, healthy hair and tight, unblemished skin rely on copper intake to stay at their best. You can get close to 250 micrograms of copper from juicing one pear.

INCREASE ENERGY

The sweetness you get from eating a pear can be a great mid-afternoon pick-me-up. When your body absorbs the glucose from a pear, it converts it into energy, leaving you with a renewed vigor to take on your day.

BETTER BREATH

One of the best side effects of eating pears is that it leaves you with fresher breath. Aside from triggering saliva in your mouth, which helps clean up the topical bacteria inside, it also helps reduce phlegm build up—a known instigator of bad breath. Really want to kick bad breath to the curb? Eat an unripe pear. They're so strong that they can even leave your mouth smelling great after eating garlic.

BUYING AND STORAGE TIPS

• Pears can be tricky to select. Your best bet is to rely on the firmness of the flesh near the stem at the top. If it has a slight give, it's good to go. If it is squishy, bruised, or pierced in any way, leave it at the store.
• If your fruit is ripe, you can store it in the fridge, making sure you don't place it near any potent foods because it will absorb scents.
• If they aren't ripe when you buy them, wrap them in a paper bag and store in a dark and dry place. But remember to move them around so they mature evenly.
• Never store pears in a plastic bag as they'll ripen too quickly and potentially damage the nutrients in the fruit.

★ = serving of green food

PEAR JUICE ★ ★ ★
1 pear, cored and chopped
1 inch (2.5 cm) fresh ginger, sliced
1 cucumber, chopped
3 stalks celery, chopped
Run all of the ingredients through a juicer.

PEAR AND CASHEW BUTTER ★
Pear slices plus cashew butter

PEAR AND WALNUT SALAD ★ ★
3 cups (60 g) baby arugula leaves
1 pear, thinly sliced
2 tablespoons (30 g) chopped walnuts, toasted
2 tablespoons (30 ml) dressing of choice
Combine the arugula, pear, and walnuts in a large bowl. Toss with dressing and serve immediately.

Easy Add-Ons to Your Diet

1. Dice pears, mangos, bell peppers, onions, and tomatoes to make a tropical salsa.
2. Cook with mixed veggies to make a stir-fry dish or soup.
3. Slice extra thin and add to raw spinach or arugula. Top with crushed walnuts, goat cheese, and a light balsamic for a great salad.
4. Purée and mix with Greek yogurt to make a great snack, dip, or dressing.
5. Add thin slices to a ham and cheese sandwich before grilling in a panini press.

PICKLES

What's better than the salty crunch you experience when you get halfway into a great burger? The pickle is reliable, savory, and perpetually considered part of the junk food empire because of how we present them in our diets. But there's a lot more to these green slices and logs than you know. For instance, pickling is a process that can happen on anything from eggs to tomatoes, but we think you'll appreciate the standard pickle the best. We do.

NUTRITIONAL INFORMATION

1 medium pickle

Calories:	12
Fat:	0.12 g
Carbohydrate:	2.68 g
Dietary fiber:	0.8 g
Sugar:	2.28 g
Protein:	0.4 g

YOU NEED TO EAT THIS

BEAT PROSTATE CANCER

Pickles contain three distinct chemical compounds called pinoresinol, lariciresinol, and secoisolariciresinol, all three of which have been proven to reduce the risk of prostate cancer.

GO CRAMP FREE

When you're working out, you're losing a lot of sweat. You're also prone to getting cramps because when you're sweating, you're burning off the salt in your system. Recent studies have found that men who drank pickle juice relieved muscle cramps almost 10 percent faster than those who drank regular water. This is because the pickle juice, and pickles by extension obviously, contain a high concentration of salt that is easily absorbed into the body. Take note though, if you've got high blood pressure, you should limit your pickle juice consumption.

CURE A HANGOVER

Hitting the bar tonight? Expecting to imbibe a little too much? Pickle juice to the rescue! Don't be so quick to dismiss this hangover cure like all the rest. Research has proven that consuming pickle juice before and after drinking can reduce hangover symptoms. The juice rehydrates you quickly by replenishing your electrolytes. Aim to drink one to two ounces (28 to 60 ml) before going out and another couple when you wake up the following morning.

STORAGE TIP

• Simple: Once you open the jar, close it up tight and refrigerate. If the water inside starts getting cloudy or the pickles start going limp or soggy, it's time for a new jar.

MEDICINE ALERT
EATING FERMENTED FOODS LIKE PICKLES WHILE TAKING PRESCRIPTION ANTIBIOTICS CREATES THE PERFECT SCENARIO FOR YOUR MEDICINE TO TAKE EFFECT AND TO HELP AVOID SIDE EFFECTS THROUGH PROPER DIGESTION.

★ = serving of green food

OVERNIGHT REFRIGERATOR PICKLES ★ ★

1 pound (455 g) small pickling cucumbers

2 cloves garlic

3 stems fresh dill

1 tablespoon (18 g) salt

2 cups (470 ml) cold water

Cut off the ends of the cucumbers and pack them tightly in a mason jar, leaving a little room at the top. Chop each clove of garlic into two or three pieces. Pack the dill and garlic in the jar. Dissolve the salt in the water and then pour the brine into the jar with the pickles. Screw on the cap and let sit at room temperature for 24 hours. Then, place the jar in the fridge and consume within the week.

MINI PICKLE SANDWICHES ★

2 ounces (55 g) deli meat (nitrate-free)

8 bread and butter pickles

Stack each piece of deli meat on top of a pickle to make mini sandwiches.

PICKLE WRAP ★ ★

4 ounces (115 g) chicken, cooked and diced

1 medium pickle

1 Swiss chard leaf

2 tablespoons (30 g) Greek yogurt

Cut a pickle in four pieces, length-wise. Lay each piece of pickle onto a Swiss chard leaf and add diced chicken breast and Greek yogurt. Add any other vegetables such as peppers, olives, and onions for taste.

GREEN ON GREEN BISON BURGER ★ ★ ★ ★

4 ounces (115 g) grass-fed bison

1 cup (67 g) kale, finely chopped

½ avocado

1 teaspoon (5 ml) coconut oil

1 dill pickle per patty

celtic salt

Put kale in a food processor (or finely chop), then sauté in coconut oil to let all the moisture out. Let cool. Add the cooled kale mixture to the ground grass-fed bison. Add a pinch of Celtic salt. Form into patties and then cool patties again. This helps because the beef fat is solid when it is cold, but at room temp it is too soft. So if cold, it will keep shape when you cook it. Once the patties are cooled, place them in pan and cook 5 to 7 minutes on each side. Top with the avocado slices and pickle.

TIP: Make the center of the patty thinner with your thumb for more even cooking.

AND ONE: Add romaine lettuce.

Easy Add-Ons to Your Diet ～～～～

1. Add to sandwiches, wraps, and salads.
2. Toss into egg salad or chicken salad dishes.
3. Add to stir-fry and pasta dishes.

PISTACHIOS

Mother Nature wants you to eat pistachios. She won't let you have them until they're ready (have you ever tried to break into an unopened pistachio?). She leaves the shells on them so your intake is regulated (meaning you'll eat less because she's slowing down your ravenous instincts). And she even packed them with essential fats, nutrients, and vitamins that you need to be your best, but she didn't skimp on the flavor. Sounds like you owe her some thanks.

NUTRITIONAL INFORMATION

1 ounce (145 g) (about 49 kernels)

Calories:	161
Fat:	13 g
Carbohydrate:	8 g
Dietary fiber:	2.8 g
Sugar:	2.2 g
Protein:	6 g

YOU NEED TO EAT THIS

SNACK LESS

People who snack on pistachios eat more than 40 percent less than those who chose other treats. Breaking open the shell and discarding it slows down your consumption and, as a result, your overall intake. Also, the fat you're getting from pistachios isn't fully absorbed by your body.

BETTER SEX

Men who ate 100 grams of pistachio each day for three weeks all showed a marked improvement in their erectile dysfunction. Eating pistachios has also shown to increase blood flow to the penis, which greatly improves erections, sexual stamina, and energy levels.

CURB CARPAL TUNNEL

Ever type so much that you find your wrists and forearms hurting? The truth is that many of us are getting carpal tunnel syndrome from our computer-obsessed culture. Some of us are getting similar pains in our hands from typing on handheld devices. To beat the pain, you need vitamin B6, and to get that you need pistachios, which are packed with the stuff.

★ = serving of green food

BOURBON MAPLE PISTACHIOS ★
8 ounces (225 g) shelled pistachios
1½ tablespoons (23 ml) bourbon
2½ tablespoons (37 ml) Grade B maple syrup
1 teaspoon (5 g) sea salt

Combine all of the ingredients together and toss well. Arrange the pistachios in a single layer on a parchment-lined baking tray, and bake for 15 minutes at 250°F (120°C or gas mark ½).

GREEN ON GREEN YOGURT PARFAIT ★ ★ ★
Layer whole-fat organic yogurt, chia pudding, or coconut yogurt with pistachios, pumpkin seeds, strawberries, and kiwi.

OATMEAL WITH PISTACHIOS ★
1 cup (80 g) oatmeal, cooked
¼ cup (35 g) green raisins, unsweetened
1 ounce (25 g) pistachios
AND ONE: Add a chopped kiwi.

ON-THE-GO LUNCH ★ ★
½ cup (75 g) pistachios
¼ cup (35 g) green raisins
3 tablespoons (45 g) shredded coconut
3 ounces (85 g) organic jerky pieces
AND ONE: Enjoy with a fresh-pressed organic green drink.

PISTACHIO-CRUSTED SALMON ★ ★
6 ounces (170 g) salmon fillet
1 cup (145 g) shelled pistachio nuts
1 tablespoon (15 ml) olive oil
2 lemons, juiced
4 tablespoons (44 g) mustard
Salt and pepper

Mix the lemon juice and mustard together and spread over the top of the salmon. Coarsely grind the pistachios in a food processer. Add the olive oil and salt and pepper, to taste. Crumbs should be slightly wet. Sprinkle the pistachio mixture over the mustard to cover the salmon evenly. Cook at 350°F (180°C or gas mark 4) for 15 to 20 minutes.

CHIA PUDDING WITH PISTACHIOS ★
Soak ⅓ cup (55 g) chia seeds in 1½ cups (355 ml) unsweetened coconut milk overnight. Sweeten with 1 tablespoon (20 g) grade B maple syrup, if necessary. Top with pistachios and kiwi.

KOMBUCHA AND PISTACHIOS ★
Kombucha and handful of pistachios

Easy Add-Ons to Your Diet
1. Use in pesto instead of pine nuts.
2. Toss into salads and trail mix for a super-powered vitamin punch.
3. Add to oatmeal or blend with some olive oil as a peanut butter alternative.

BUYING AND STORAGE TIPS
• Unshelled nuts may be stored for three months in the refrigerator or up to one year in the freezer.
• Shelled pistachios can be stored in the refrigerator for up to three months but are not a good candidate for freezing.
• We recommend buying the ones with shells so you snack a little slower. Also, avoid any that have been salted to limit your salt intake. Pass on the roasted variety as they've lost much of their vitamin content.

PUMPKIN SEEDS

You know all that stuff you threw out when you were making jack-o'-lanterns? Well, it turns out those guts had more value than you think. Pumpkin seeds are a great, sensible snack that pack a serious healthy punch for men of all ages and all fitness levels. Get some. You and your wife will thank us later.

NUTRITIONAL INFORMATION

½ cup (70 g)

Calories:	143
Fat:	6 g
Carbohydrate:	17 g
Dietary fiber:	6 g
Sugar:	0 g
Protein:	6 g

YOU NEED TO EAT THIS

BOOST YOUR TESTOSTERONE

Boost your testosterone by eating a diet that contains the zinc-supercharged pumpkin seed. Low zinc levels increase your chances of impotency, enlarged prostate, and a myriad of other sexual health issues. Snacking on pumpkin seeds gives you the zinc your body needs, which will bring you back to your best, increase sperm motility and sperm count, and even help prevent prostate issues.

LIVE LONGER

If you want to live longer, you need to eat pumpkin seeds. Recent research indicates that men who have higher levels of magnesium in their blood have a 40 percent lower risk of dying early. Guys with low magnesium kicked the bucket long before their time.

SLEEP BETTER

Tryptophan is your friend. Your body converts this amino acid into serotonin and then again into the sleep inducing hormone, melatonin. This process is how you get a good night's sleep. Pumpkin seeds are a rich source of tryptophan, which means they're your key to better sleep.

STORAGE TIPS

• Store your pumpkin seeds in an airtight container in your freezer (up to six months) or in your cupboard. Just be sure to keep them sealed up tight, as they can go bad quick when exposed to the air. You'll know they have gone rancid because they will smell "off," almost like paint.

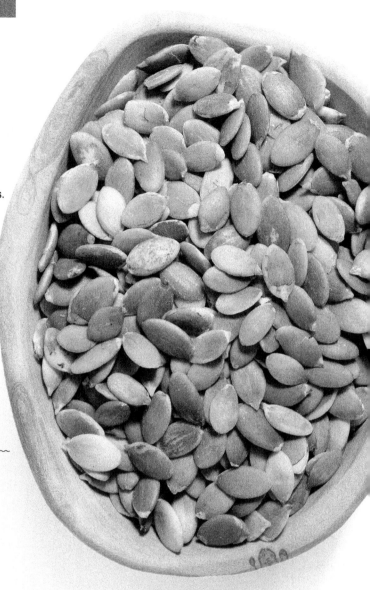

★ = serving of green food

PUMPKIN SEED BREADCRUMBS ★ ★

1 cup (64 g) roasted pumpkin seeds

½ clove fresh garlic

1 teaspoon (5 g) lemon zest

Sea salt

2 leaves fresh basil

Grind all of the ingredients in a food processor for a gluten-free version of breadcrumbs to coat your chicken or fish before grilling and baking. Dip the chicken or fish in whisked egg first, so the coating sticks.

POWER-UP SMOOTHIE ★ ★ ★

½ avocado

1 tablespoon (15 g) pumpkin seeds, raw

2 cups (60 g) spinach

1 medium banana

2 teaspoons (10 g) raw honey

12 ounces (355 ml) water

Blend all of the ingredients until smooth.

SPROUTED PUMPKIN SEEDS ★

Soaked and sprouted pumpkin seeds

Easy Add-Ons to Your Diet

1. Add to guacamole to add a crunch.
2. Roast on a pan with some sea salt to make a great snack.
3. Add to oatmeal and trail mix.

ROMAINE LETTUCE

When you think of salad, you're probably imagining a bowl of some sad light green lettuce that's been chopped up and plated with just a few carrot shavings on top as garnish. No wonder you hate the stuff! Well, that salad is definitely boring and we don't think you should eat it. Instead of the tired old iceberg lettuce salad, we're suggesting you reach for the romaine. It has a better crunch, more flavor, and a hell of a lot more nutrients per serving.

NUTRITIONAL INFORMATION

1 cup (55 g)

Calories:	8
Fat:	0.1 g
Carbohydrate:	1.6 g
Dietary fiber:	1 g
Sugar:	0 g
Protein:	0.6 g

YOU NEED TO EAT THIS

SLEEP BETTER

You know that milky substance in romaine lettuce? Turns out it's lettuce latex and it could be a major difference maker in how well you sleep. Doctors suggest that ingesting lettuce juice before bedtime could help you get a better night's sleep and even act as a pain reliever.

BEAT IMPOTENCE

Just when you thought eating lettuce was only done in emergencies, some studies have shown that consuming large amounts of romaine can actually prevent impotence. Researchers are still working on the reasons why, but if you find yourself needing an edge, romaine could be your secret weapon.

BE YOUR BEST

Want to know what else romaine can help you with? Well, how about boosting your metabolism, priming your muscle growth, beating bad breath, helping your skin look healthier and younger, and making sure you've got a full head of great hair? Good enough for you?

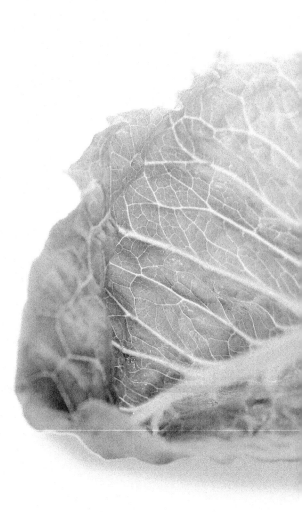

★ = serving of green food

GRILLED ROMAINE AND PROSCIUTTO ★ ★

½ head of romaine lettuce

2 slices thin prosciutto

1 tablespoon (15 ml) coconut oil

Salt and pepper

Your favorite vinegar

Wash and slice the heads of the romaine lengthwise. Glaze with the coconut oil, vinegar, salt, and pepper. Wrap with prosciutto. Grill hot and fast.

ROMAINE AND CARROT JUICE ★ ★

1 head of romaine

5 carrots

Process the ingredients through a juicer.

Easy Add-Ons to Your Diet

1. Use instead of a bread wrap to limit refined carb intake.
2. Use as a dipper or as the dipping bowl.
3. Chop and serve with other mixed greens to make a salad.
4. Drizzle olive oil on top and grill with seasoning of choice and serve with shaved Parmesan.
5. Juice romaine whole and mix with lime juice and mango for a tropical drink.

STORAGE TIPS

• Snap off all of the leaves and rinse in cold water. Pat dry and serve full or chopped.
• You can refrigerate romaine in a plastic bag for about a week.

ROSEMARY

It's entirely possible that you've never noticed rosemary. But that's kind of why it's so important. It's like a secret squad of Navy Seals that infiltrate your meals and infuse them with flavor and nutrients, but you don't even notice before it's too late. Rosemary might just be the unsung hero of your wife's herb garden, but so long as you're enjoying the taste and health benefits, it's fine with that.

NUTRITIONAL INFORMATION

1 tablespoon (1.7 g), fresh

Calories:	2
Fat:	0.1 g
Carbohydrate:	0.4 g
Dietary fiber:	0.2 g
Sugar:	0 g
Protein:	0.1 g

YOU NEED TO EAT THIS

MENTAL CLARITY
Recent research has discovered that just smelling rosemary can improve your mental capacity. Further studies have proven that the essential oils in rosemary greatly increase mental clarity primarily because of how it boosts circulation. It even sharpens your memory.

BEAT HAIR LOSS
An age-old solution for an age-old problem: hair loss. Massaging rosemary oil on the scalp has been proven to help men grow new hair. But you don't have to tell anyone you're using it for hair loss—you can also use rosemary oil on sore muscles, too.

STRESS LESS
Rosemary oil can also lower your cortisol levels, ultimately reducing your anxiety and bringing about a calmer state. Ancient Greeks wore rosemary in their hair during test taking to improve their energy levels and squash any stress.

COOK SMARTER
Cooking animal flesh creates cancer-causing compounds called heterocyclic amines. Researchers have recently discovered that adding rosemary to the meats during cooking helped prevent these ill effects from happening.

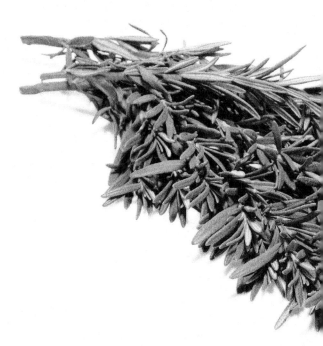

STORAGE TIPS
• You can store fresh rosemary in a plastic bag or a glass of water in your fridge.
• If you're storing dried rosemary, take the leaves off the stems and store in an airtight container in your cupboard.

★ = serving of green food

NATURE'S CHILL PILL ★ ★

1 fresh banana

½ cup (75 g) frozen blueberries

1 cup (30 g) spinach

2 sprigs fresh rosemary, leaves removed and finely chopped

1 to 2 cups (235 to 475 ml) water

Dash of Celtic sea salt

A little raw honey or maple syrup to sweeten

Blend all of the ingredients on high, until smooth.

ROSEMARY BEETS MARINATED IN OLIVE OIL ★

1 cup (225 g) cooked beets

1 tablespoon (1.7 g) rosemary, chopped

3 tablespoons (45 ml) olive oil

Drizzle olive oil over the beets and sprinkle with rosemary.

HERB-ROASTED SQUASH ★

1 cup (255 g) butternut squash, cubed

1 tablespoon (1.7 g) rosemary, chopped

1 clove garlic, minced

1 tablespoon (15 ml) coconut oil, melted

Salt and pepper

Roast squash on a lined baking sheet at 400°F (200°C, gas mark 6) for 30 minutes, until squash is lightly browned and tender. Toss the squash cubes with rosemary, garlic, salt, pepper, and coconut oil.

Easy Add-Ons to Your Diet

1. Add to protein sources for flavor.
2. Include in dry rubs or marinades.
3. Add to soups or Greek yogurt to make a dip.

SAGE

Sage is another ubiquitous leaf that's full of health benefits, but you're probably a little weary of it. We understand that. But what if we told you sage is one of the only reasons you're so in love with your fattier meats? You know that exotic flavor you get when you're chowing down on a pork chop? That flavor you're liking is probably sage. Try it in some other dishes and we bet you'll reach for the fattier dishes a little less and the sage seasoning a little more.

NUTRITIONAL INFORMATION

1 tablespoon (2.5 g)

Calories:	6
Fat:	0.3 g
Carbohydrate:	1.2 g
Dietary fiber:	1 g
Sugar:	0 g
Protein:	0.2 g

YOU NEED TO EAT THIS

MENTAL HEALTH

If there's one thing you should consume to protect and strengthen your brain, it's sage. Recent research has proven that it can reduce depression. College students who took sage extract reported improved memory when taking tests. Sage can also help with word recall so you won't ever have to suffer through someone else finishing your sentences.

CURE THE COMMON COLD

Feeling a little under the weather? Sage has been proven to aid in the detoxification process and can even help you beat a fever. It also purifies your blood, so you're healthier from the inside out. Sage tea is a common sore throat reliever, too.

STOMACH PAIN RELIEVER

Your stomach loves sage. It doesn't matter if you've lost your appetite or are overeating, have too much gas or cramps, or are suffering from diarrhea, bloating, or a simple upset stomach, sage in your diet or sipping sage tea is your answer.

STORAGE TIPS

• Wrap your sage leaves in a paper towel and store them in the fridge, locked in an airtight bag. They'll last for almost a week. If you want them to last longer, submerge them in olive oil and they'll be good for about a month.
• If you want to freeze it, remove the leaves from the stems and store in an airtight bag. This will keep them fresh for a year.
• Keep dried sage in an airtight jar and store it in a dark cupboard.

★ = serving of green food

SAGE EGGS ★

2 eggs

2 teaspoons (20 ml) coconut oil

2 sage leaves

In a pan, heat the coconut oil, add the sage leaves, and cook until they start to brown. Reduce heat, add egg mixture, and gently stir to scramble and cook until golden.

Easy Add-Ons to Your Diet

1. Add to fattier protein sources like lamb and pork.
2. Sprinkle over egg scrambles.
3. Add chopped fresh leaves or dried leaves and lime juice to Greek yogurt to make a dip.

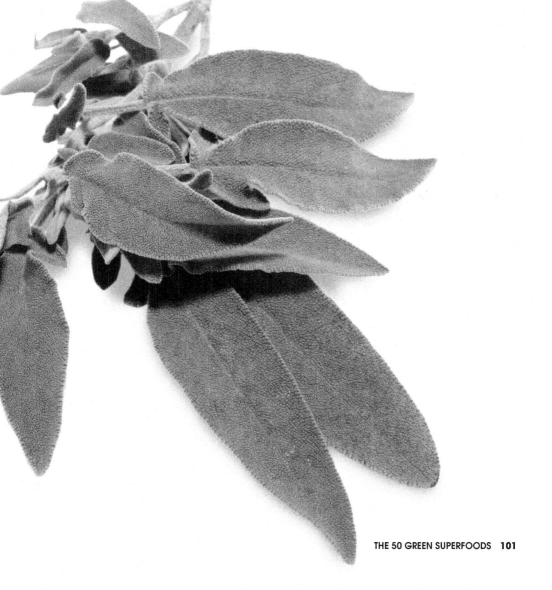

SAUERKRAUT

You've probably already had fermented cabbage, a.k.a. sauerkraut, on a ballpark hotdog. When a food is fermented, the yeast, bacteria, or mold used to do this predigests the foods and creates probiotics (good bacteria needed to maintain healthy digestion and keep your immune system strong). What does this mean for you? Well, the next time your wife starts raving about her yogurt being packed with probiotics, you can tell her you're way ahead of her. If you really want to impress her and benefit from all the good stuff in fermented cabbage, we've even included a plan on how to do it yourself so you can look smarter and reap all the rewards as well.

NUTRITIONAL INFORMATION

½ cup (142 g)

Calories:	14
Fat:	0.1 g
Carbohydrate:	3 g
Dietary fiber:	2 g
Sugar:	1 g
Protein:	0.7 g

YOU NEED TO EAT THIS

HAVE BETTER HAIR AND SKIN AND BEAT STRESS

Under a lot of pressure lately? Have you counted a few more follicles hitting the bathroom floor every morning than usual? Is your skin inflamed? These are symptoms of stress. Eating a healthy diet including sauerkraut can combat the symptoms and the cause.

BUST STOMACH PAIN

Ingesting fermented cabbage has been proven to help in most stomach ailments, including protecting against salmonella, E. coli, and high amounts of candida, as well as calm the symptoms of lactose intolerance. It has also been proven to help with the common upset stomach or constipation and even combat colon cancer and ulcers.

REDUCE CHOLESTEROL

Cabbage binds the bile in your intestine, allowing it to stay there and only pass via a bowel movement instead of getting absorbed during the process. This then triggers your liver to create new bile by using your already existing cholesterol, thus dropping your levels in the process.

Easy Add-Ons to Your Diet

1. Add to potato salad or coleslaw.
2. Mix into soups for a flavor boost.
3. Add to roasted protein sources and let caramelize in the pan to suck in some flavor from the roasting process.
4. Before you shred it and ferment it, take off larger leafs and use them as wraps for burgers.
5. Add to meatballs before cooking for a tangy flavor kick.

BUYING TIPS

• Don't get lazy and buy canned sauerkraut. The canned stuff not only contains a harmful chemical in the lining of the can called bisphenol-A, but it's also been pasteurized, which negates the super-powered probiotics that you get when you make it yourself.

☆ = serving of green food

HOMEMADE SAUERKRAUT ☆

1 head cabbage, shredded

1 tablespoon (18 g) sea salt

3 cups (700 ml) water plus more to cover cabbage

Mix the salt and cabbage in a non-metal bowl with a wooden spoon. Let the mixture sit for 1 to 2 hours so juices form. Pack tightly into two sterilized quart size mason jars. Push the cabbage down so juices cover it. Add 1 cup (235 ml) of water and 1 teaspoon (5 g) of salt at a time. Continue to add until cabbage is covered with liquid.

Cover the jar loosely with a lid. Each day push down the mixture with a wooden spoon to make sure the cabbage stays immersed. If the water falls below the cabbage, add a bit more salt water. Let the mixture sit for 2 to 4 weeks or until it stops bubbling. Refrigerate. (It is important that you don't refrigerate the sauerkraut for at least 10 days.)

NOTE: If the sauerkraut is brown or pink, has a yeasty odor, or has mold, do not use it. It's fine if it appears cloudy, but any other colors suggest yeast or mold overgrowth. Do not eat it in this state!

SAUER-SLAW ☆ ☆

2 cups (280 g) sauerkraut

1 small carrot, grated

2 tablespoons (30 ml) olive oil

1 teaspoon (5 ml) raw honey

Mix together all of the ingredients.

BRAISED SAUERKRAUT WITH BRATWURST SAUSAGE ☆

1 cup (142 g) sauerkraut

½ onion, diced

1 apple, sliced thinly

2 tablespoons (22 g) Dijon or whole grain mustard

4 ounces (115 g) Bratwurst sausage (nitrate-free), cooked

Braise the drained sauerkraut in a pan with onions and thin apple slices. Add the sausage slices and warm. After cooking, mix in mustard and serve.

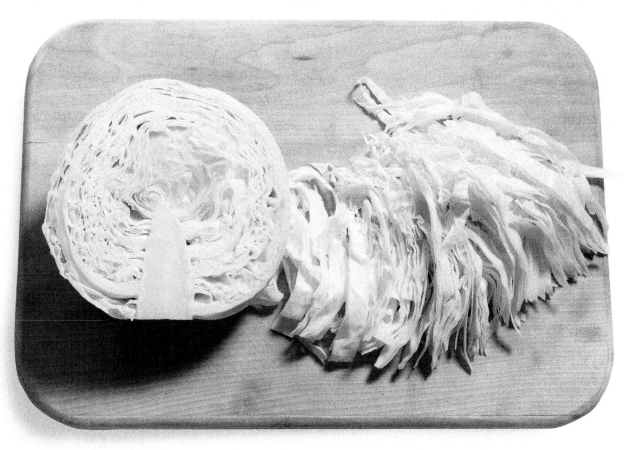

SEAWEED

Pulling seaweed from the ocean may have been considered insane at one point in time, but it sure seems like genius today, and not just because they use it in sushi. Sea plants contain up to twenty times the minerals of the stuff growing on dry land and in some instances, like with seaweed, they're great sources of hard-to-get but vital substances like iodine. Overall, seaweed provides you with fifty-six minerals and trace minerals, often packing a serious punch (ten times the calcium of milk and more iron than red meat). And if you find yourself at sea, it also acts as a remedy for seasickness. That's convenient.

NUTRITIONAL INFORMATION

2 tablespoons or 1 ounce (30 g)
(fresh kelp)

Calories:	4
Fat:	0.1 g
Carbohydrate:	0 g
Dietary fiber:	0.1 g
Sugar:	0.1 g
Protein:	0.2 g

YOU NEED TO EAT THIS

HOTTER SEX

All four classes of seaweed (green, red, brown, and blue green) have high manganese content, which makes them an aphrodisiac for men. As well, because seaweed is high in vitamin E, it also helps you produce healthier sperm.

BALANCE HORMONES

If you've ever told your wife she was acting weird because of hormones, you've probably been slapped a few times. We can't help with the spankings, but we can tell you that you've got hormones and they need regulating as well. Seaweed is high in iodine, which is rare in most foods and is vital to making your thyroid work properly—ultimately ensuring your body is running right in the hormone department. Trust in the seaweed to help you with fatigue, bad memory, heart issues, high cholesterol, and feelings of weakness in all your muscles.

STAY LEAN

Been working out a lot lately? If you have, then you're low on a vital element to get lean: salt. Since you've been doing your best to sweat off the pounds—and losing salt in the process—replenish your sodium and fire up your metabolism with seaweed.

BEAN SECRET
ADD SOME SEAWEED TO YOUR BEANS WHEN COOKING. JUST BY INCLUDING IT IN THE POT, IT'LL REDUCE RAFFINOSE IN THE BEANS, WHICH IS THE CARB THAT PRODUCES GAS IN BEANS.

★ = serving of green food

DULSE MISO SOUP ★ ★

2 cups (475 ml) boiling water

1 tablespoon (15 g) miso

¼ cup (55 g) sliced dulse seaweed

2 tablespoons (30 g) minced green onion

1 tablespoon (8 g) grated ginger

Add all of the ingredients to boiling water. Simmer for 7 minutes or until seaweed is tender.

SEAWEED SALAD ★ ★

2 ounces (60 g) wakame dried and cut seaweed

1 teaspoon (2 g) fresh minced ginger

1 teaspoon (3 g) fresh minced garlic

1 teaspoon (5 ml) white wine vinegar

2 teaspoons (10 ml) toasted sesame oil

¼ teaspoon raw honey

Soak the seaweed in warm water to cover, 5 minutes. Drain and blot excess water with a paper towel. Whisk together the garlic, ginger, vinegar, sesame oil, and honey. Drizzle on top of the seaweed and toss to coat.

Easy Add-Ons to Your Diet

1. Add to steamed veggies or soups.
2. Include in your green smoothies (kelp powder or dulse flakes work best).
3. Add dried flakes to rice dishes and egg scrambles.

STORAGE TIP

• Dry seaweed will last for almost half a year in your fridge, if you keep it in a sealed container. If you store it in your cupboard, it'll go bad in about four months. Want to rehydrate your seaweed? This can easily be done with some fresh water, but beware because it'll go bad in a few days.

SPINACH

Popeye may have made this green popular, but you're going to be the guy who benefits most from all the healthy goodness it provides. Why? Because you're going to look past the unhealthy spinach dip at your local pub and eat this stuff in spite of the fact that you've scoffed at it before. And when you do, you'll not only be ready to take on Bluto, but you'll have more than enough energy to spend time with Olive as well.

NUTRITIONAL INFORMATION

1 cup (30 g)

Calories:	7
Fat:	0.1 g
Carbohydrate:	1.1 g
Dietary fiber:	0.7 g
Sugar:	0.1 g
Protein:	0.9 g

YOU NEED TO EAT THIS

BOOST TESTOSTERONE NATURALLY

Calcium from cooked spinach may be the key to naturally spiking your testosterone. Researchers have discovered that men who supplement with calcium had higher levels of free testosterone after their workouts than those who didn't have a high calcium diet plan.

GET HAPPY

Optimistic people have higher levels of carotenoids, which are plant pigments from spinach, kale, and squash. Recent research indicates that men who ate at least three servings daily of foods that were high in carotenoids were happier than their counterparts who didn't consume comparable fare.

BUILD MORE MUSCLE

Studies indicate that spinach contains a muscle-building and repairing hormone. Furthermore, researchers have discovered that high-nitrate foods like spinach can cause the protein in your system to trigger the calcium in your blood to make you have stronger contractions, which means you'll have a more productive, muscle-building workout.

BOIL = BEST
YOUR BEST COOKING METHOD IS BOILING, WHICH ENSURES THE MOST AMOUNT OF NUTRIENTS STAY IN THE LEAVES.

Easy Add-Ons to Your Diet

1. Blend into Greek yogurt and add some leeks for a savory spinach dip.
2. Include in egg and pasta dishes.
3. Fillet chicken breast and fold in some spinach leaves and organic cheese before cooking.
4. Include in your green salads.
5. Include in soups and smoothies.

STORAGE AND PREP TIPS

• Raw spinach can last for almost a week in your fridge, if it's wrapped in a damp towel and bagged with an airtight seal.
• Make sure you wait to wash your spinach to just before you're about to eat it so it'll last longer.

★ = serving of green food

SPINBERRY SMOOTHIE ★ ★ ★

3 cups (90 g) spinach, fresh

½ cup (75 g) frozen strawberries

Juice of half lemon

2 teaspoons (10 g) raw honey

10 ounces (285 ml) water (less for thicker smoothie, more for thinner smoothie)

Blend all of the ingredients until smooth.

PRE-WORKOUT BOOSTER ★

1 cup (30 g) spinach, fresh

1 cup (235 ml) water

1 cup (165 g) pineapple, fresh or frozen

½ banana

4 unsweetened coconut milk ice cubes

Blend all of the ingredients until smooth.

SWEET GREEN SCRAMBLE ★ ★ ★

1 sweet potato, chopped

3 eggs

1 cup (67 g) kale, chopped

1 tablespoon (15 ml) coconut oil

½ avocado

½ cup (15 g) spinach

Heat a pan and coat it with coconut oil. Chop up the sweet potato into slices and mix it into the pan. Cover and cook for 3 to 4 minutes or until half cooked. Cut up the kale and add it to the pan and mix it up with the sweet potatoes. Cover for 1 minute. Crack 3 eggs into the pan and scramble together with the kale and sweet potatoes. Cook until desired readiness and serve atop a bed of spinach, garnished with a half or one whole avocado, sliced.

SPIRULINA

Everything in this book up to this point hasn't really scared you, right? Maybe a mysterious powder with an odd-sounding name might do the trick. Spirulina (that's not a typo or a translation of someone's last name) is a form of blue-green algae that only grows in fresh bodies of water. Temperature and adverse weather conditions don't seem to stop it from thriving, and it's been considered as a legitimate solution to end world hunger. It's got more protein than your steak, more nutrients than just about anything you've ever eaten, and should be on your shopping list.

NUTRITIONAL INFORMATION

1 tablespoon (15 g), dried

Calories:	20
Fat:	1 g
Carbohydrate:	2 g
Dietary fiber:	0 g
Sugar:	0 g
Protein:	4 g

YOU NEED TO EAT THIS

BETTER PROTEIN

You need your protein to feed your muscles. That's why you eat lean meats and supplement with protein powder. But meat only has 27 percent protein on average, while spirulina is a more pure source, composed of 60 percent protein.

STAY YOUNG

Slow down aging with the spirulina triple threat: vitamin E, selenium, and tyrosine. All three are integral in making you healthier, but research shows that they are also vital to keeping you virile a lot longer.

SNACK LESS

You can curb your cravings by supplementing with spirulina. It's not just a great protein source, which will keep you fuller longer, but it's also packed with more than one hundred nutrients that ensure you're not in a state where you'll need or want to reach for anything else.

LAST LONGER

Recent research is favorably reporting that spirulina can also help your endurance and postpone exhaustion. While more research is needed to really be sure of this process, the study subjects who took the spirulina all reported more favorable conditions than those who didn't.

STORAGE TIP

• Dried spirulina can last in an airtight container in your cupboard for more than six months.

★ = serving of green food

QUICK BREAKFAST SMOOTHIE ★ ★

2 cups (60 g) spinach

1 cup (150 g) frozen fruit

1 to 2 scoops protein powder

1 cup (235 ml) coconut milk

1 teaspoon (5 g) spirulina

Blend all of the ingredients into a smoothie.

ENERGY BALLS ★

2 cups (270 g) raw cashews

1 cup (178 g) dates (pre-soaked for five minutes, drained)

1 tablespoon (15 ml) coconut oil

1 tablespoon (20 g) raw honey

1 tablespoon (15 g) spirulina

1/8 teaspoon unrefined sea salt

1 cup (80 g) unsweetened coconut shreds

Place the raw cashews in a food processor and chop relatively fine. Remove the pits from the dates and process until well blended. Add the coconut oil, raw honey, spirulina, and sea salt. Blend until well combined. Measure out ping-pong ball size scoops and roll in the unsweetened coconut shreds. Cool in the fridge so they harden. Keep in fridge.

Easy Add-Ons to Your Diet

1. Blend into smoothies.
2. Include in pancake mixes for a protein punch.
3. Mix into yogurt or pudding to add flavor and protein.

SWISS CHARD

This tall leafy green comes with various colorful stocks, including purple, yellow, and orange. The leaves are super-powered with vital nutrients and minerals—more than most foods you're eating. No wonder it's a staple of the healthiest Mediterranean diets.

NUTRITIONAL INFORMATION

1 cup (30 g)

Calories:	7
Fat:	0.1 g
Carbohydrate:	1.4 g
Dietary fiber:	0.6 g
Sugar:	0.4 g
Protein:	0.6 g

YOU NEED TO EAT THIS

LOWER BLOOD PRESSURE

Swiss chard is a great source of magnesium, which has become a proven tool to help keep blood pressure at healthy levels. With one out of every three adults in the U.S. alone having high blood pressure, and men having higher risk levels than women for most age groups, reaching for some Swiss chard just got a lot more necessary.

HANGOVER AND HEADACHE CURE

Maybe you had too much to drink last night, or maybe you're one of millions of American men who suffer from migraines, or maybe both. Bottom line: A diet rich in foods like Swiss chard has been proven to help ease migraines and prevent the pain in your skull after drinking a little too much.

BOOST TESTOSTERONE

Loaded with zinc, Swiss chard might be the answer you need to keep your prostate functioning in perfect order. It's also been proven to help naturally boost your testosterone.

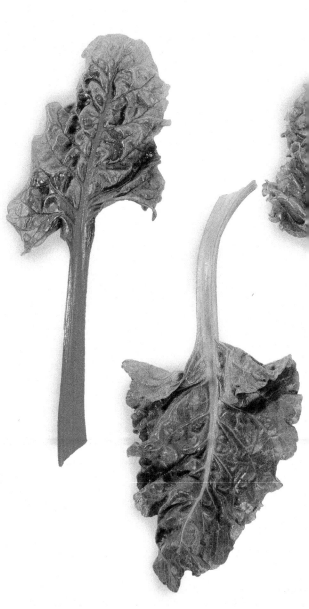

★ = serving of green food

BALSAMIC CHARD ★ ★

2 cups (60 g) Swiss chard

1 tablespoon (15 ml) balsamic vinegar

Salt

Steam the Swiss chard. Drizzle it with balsamic vinegar and add salt to taste.

CHICKEN AND CHARD BOWL ★ ★

½ cup (70 g) shredded cooked chicken

½ onion, chopped

2 cloves garlic

2 cups (60 g) Swiss chard, destemmed and chopped

2 tablespoons (30 ml) coconut oil

Heat the coconut oil, add the onions and cook until soft. Add garlic and chicken and cook for an additional few minutes. Add the Swiss chard to the pan and cook while stirring frequently. Cook for approximately 5 minutes or until chard is soft.

Easy Add-Ons to Your Diet

1. Chop and add to salads.
2. Sauté with other veggies and serve as a side or base to your main.
3. Use leaf as a wrap for meatballs or other ground meats.

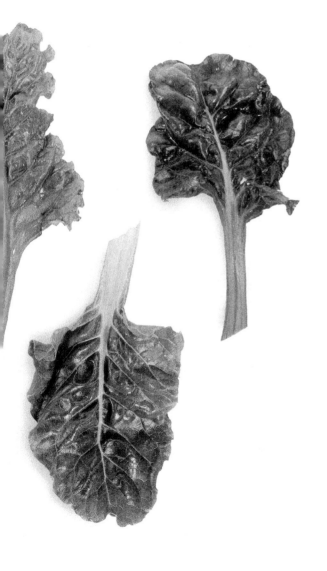

PREP TIP

• The colorful stems of this leafy green actually don't cook well. As such, we suggest removing them before cooking them—steaming being the best option to retain as many vitamins as possible.

STORAGE TIP

• When you store your Swiss chard, put them in a tightly sealed bag and leave in the fridge, but don't wash first. It'll keep for about a week.

THYME

Ancient Egyptians used thyme to embalm their dead. Ancient Greeks considered it a symbol of courage and burned it like incense. In the sixteenth century, it was used as a mouthwash. You know what all of these eras had in common? They knew thyme was extremely healthy, very versatile, and had potential even if they weren't quite sure how to maximize its effectiveness. Now we know that thyme can help you live longer and be healthier than you ever dreamed.

NUTRITIONAL INFORMATION

1 teaspoon (0.8 g)

Calories:	1
Fat:	0 g
Carbohydrate:	0.2 g
Dietary fiber:	0.1 g
Sugar:	0 g
Protein:	0.04 g

YOU NEED TO EAT THIS

HEALTHY CELLS

Best known for being a superior anti-inflammatory, thyme helps protect your cell membranes because it contains thymol. This substance can be integral to safeguarding your heart, kidneys, brain, and blood cells from damage.

STAY HEALTHY

Thyme is so powerful that it can even kill bacteria like staphylococcus. It may also protect you from chest congestion, bronchitis, and coughs.

MORE ENERGY, LESS FAT

Ever think something so unassuming could be a stimulant? Probably not. Thyme, however, is a solid alternative to other more potentially harmful energy boosters because it stimulates your entire system, including your metabolism.

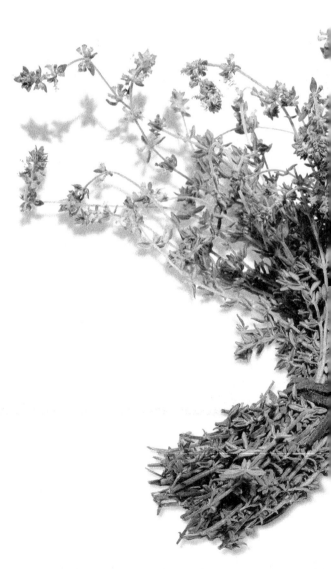

BUYING AND STORAGE TIPS

• Fresh thyme is always a better option over the dried variety. Your best bet is to look for the greenish-gray colored leaves that have no spots or yellowing.
• Wrap them in a damp paper towel and refrigerate them in an airtight container.
• If you go with dried thyme, keep it in an airtight jar, and it'll stay healthy for six months.

★ = serving of green food

LEMON THYME MUSHROOMS ★

2 cups (140 g) sliced button mushrooms

3 springs fresh thyme, leaves only

1 garlic clove, diced

Zest of 1 lemon

1 tablespoon (15 ml) coconut oil

Salt and pepper

Heat the coconut oil in a pan. Add the mushrooms and thyme until browned. Then add the garlic, lemon zest, salt, and pepper. Cook until mushrooms are tender. Garnish with fresh lemon juice and more fresh thyme.

THYME TEA ★

2 tablespoons (4.8 g) fresh thyme (or 1 tablespoon (4.3 g) of dried)

2 tablespoons (20 g) raw honey (optional)

Steep the thyme in hot water for 10 minutes. Add the raw honey, if needed. Optional add-ins include ginger, lemon juice, turmeric, and cayenne pepper. This works as an excellent remedy for a cough or sore throat.

LEMON THYME FISH HOT POCKET ★ ★ ★

4 to 6 ounces (115 to 165 g) white mild fish

Lemon juice

1 tablespoon (2.4 g) thyme

½ cup (150 g) fennel, coarsely chopped

½ cup (60 g) zucchini, coarsely chopped

2 tablespoons (30 ml) coconut oil

Cut some parchment paper so it is about 18 inches (46 cm) wide and fold it in half. Keeping the paper folded, use kitchen scissors to cut it into a heart shape. Fill half the heart with all of your ingredients. Fold the edges of the parchment paper so it creates a sealed pocket. Place this on a baking sheet and bake for 12 to 15 minutes at 350°F (180°C or gas mark 4). (If frozen vegetables, add 3 minutes). Pull from the oven and let rest for 3 to 5 minutes. Carefully open pocket. Fish is done when it flakes easily with a fork.

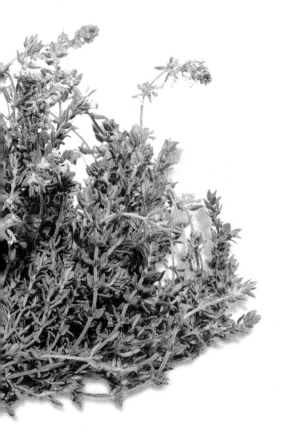

Easy Add-Ons to Your Diet

1. Chop and toss into salads or add to yogurt or olive oil to make your own dressing.
2. Add to pasta sauces and egg scrambles.
3. Use to season protein while cooking or include in a dry rub or marinade before cooking.

TOMATILLOS

Looks a little like an unripe tomato? We know. But trust us when we tell you that this green guy is ready to eat just as he is. Often overlooked in the search for a spice in your home because it never made it past the front door, tomatillos are what make green salsa spicy, tart, and peppery. We suggest you include it in your quest to add veggies to your diet. It'll taste great and help you live longer. Sounds like a good suggestion, doesn't it?

NUTRITIONAL INFORMATION

1 medium	
Calories:	11
Fat:	0 g
Carbohydrate:	2 g
Dietary fiber:	1 g
Sugar:	1 g
Protein:	0.3 g

YOU NEED TO EAT THIS

GET LEAN
Eating one cup of tomatillo equals only 2 percent of your daily recommended allowance of calories per day. Why is this important? Because it's low in calories, but high on flavor. That means you'll get to eat a lot of a tasty veggie without any possible harm to your waistline.

HEALTHIER SKIN, HEALTHIER YOU
One serving of tomatillo gives you 26 percent of your daily recommended allowance of vitamin C, which you've no doubt heard will keep cold and flu symptoms at bay. But, that's not all. It'll also trigger the production of white blood cells and collagen. All of this will help your skin look better and leave you feeling bulletproof from just about any ailment.

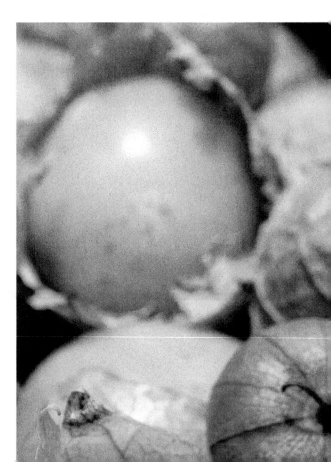

TASTES

☆ = serving of green food

TOMATILLO SALSA VERDE ☆ ☆ ☆

2 cups (360 g) tomatillos, destemmed

3 jalapeños

2 garlic cloves

1 medium onion

⅓ cup (5 g) fresh cilantro

Salt to taste

Combine all of the ingredients in a food processor and blend. Add water to achieve desired texture.

TOMATILLO SMOOTHIE ☆ ☆ ☆ ☆

1 cup tomatillos (180 g), chopped

1 medium cucumber, peeled and chopped

1 jalapeño, seeded and chopped

¾ cup (175 ml) water

3 tablespoons (45 ml) fresh lime juice

1 tablespoon (20 g) raw honey

½ teaspoon salt

Pinch cayenne pepper

Blend all of the ingredients until smooth.

Easy Add-Ons to Your Diet

1. Chop and toss into salsa verde, pico de gallo, and guacamole.
2. Add to tacos, wraps, and stir-fry dishes.
3. Purée and add to yogurt with some lime juice to make a great dressing or dip.

PREP TIP

• Remove the husk of your tomatillo before cooking. They'll usually pop right out if you squeeze gently at the base of the husk. Once they're out, they can be a little sticky so try running it under cold water. From there, use them as your recipe calls for it.

STORAGE TIP

• We suggest freezing them whole in an airtight bag.

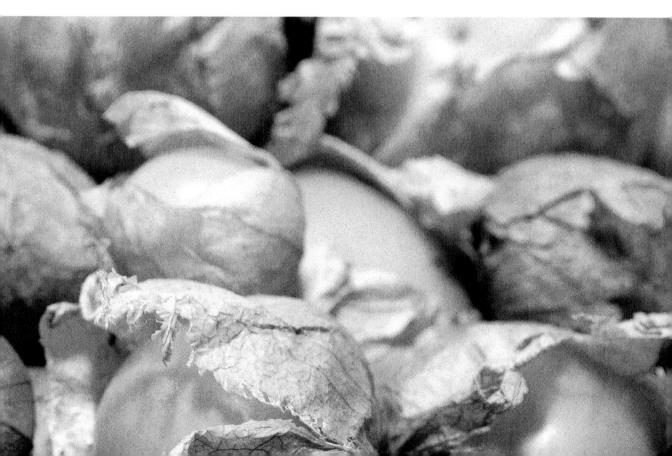

TURNIP GREENS

You may think we're asking you to eat the leftover portion of this veggie, but the truth is that turnip greens really pack a powerful health punch. Popular in ancient Europe, these greens became a dietary fixture in the southern U.S. during the era of slavery. Slave owners discarded the leaves in favor of eating just the turnip. The slaves, however, took to including the greens in their diet and reaped the healthy rewards. While not the most versatile green in this book, it definitely deserves your attention.

NUTRITIONAL INFORMATION

1 cup (150 g), chopped

Calories:	18
Fat:	0.16 g
Carbohydrate:	3.92 g
Dietary fiber:	1.8 g
Sugar:	0.45 g
Protein:	0.82 g

YOU NEED TO EAT THIS

BETTER SEX

As an excellent source of folate, a diet rich in turnip greens lowers homocysteine levels in your body, which can cause damage to your arteries and slow blood flow. Eliminating this problem keeps your blood circulating at optimum conditions, and that means better blood flow throughout your body—especially in your extremities, which means you'll have better erections.

BEAT ULCERS

Lots of guys are walking around with a pain in their gut. Many of them are suffering from ulcers caused by *H. Pylori*, which can also trigger colon cancer and a myriad of other health concerns. Turnip greens contain glucoraphanin and sulforaphane, which can outright kill *H. Pylori* and protect your gut better than body armor.

STAY REGULAR

With five grams of quality fiber in each cup, turnip greens can help your digestive tract stay on track. Because of this, it will also help prevent constipation and other stomach-related disorders.

RINSE, SOAK, ENJOY
BEFORE COOKING, RINSE THOROUGHLY AND THEN LET THEM SIT IN SOME WATER FOR FIVE MINUTES. THIS WILL ACTUALLY HELP ENZYMES IN THE GREENS COMPOUND, RESULTING IN EVEN MORE NUTRIENTS AND BENEFITS.

STORAGE TIPS

• When you get your turnip greens home, you should cut the turnip off and store the greens separately.
• All you need is an airtight bag and they'll stay fresh in your fridge for about four days.

★ = serving of green food

DIJON TURNIP GREENS ★ ★

2 cups (300 g) turnip greens, chopped

1 tablespoon (11 g) Dijon mustard

2 teaspoons (10 ml) coconut oil

Sauté the greens in coconut oil. Remove from heat and stir in the Dijon mustard for a tangy side dish.

TURNIP GREEN SMOOTHIE ★ ★ ★

1 cup (150 g) turnip greens

¼ head green cabbage

1 green apple, cored

1 orange, juiced

Juice the orange first. Combine it with the greens, cabbage, and apple. Blend all of the ingredients until smooth. Add water or ice if needed for desired consistency.

Easy Add-Ons to Your Diet

1. Boil and top with sautéed veggies.
2. Add to juices and smoothies.
3. Mix and serve with fermented cabbage to add color and nutrients.

ZUCCHINI

This little Italian green may look, taste, and be most often prepared as a vegetable, but it is actually a fruit. It is cousins with the pumpkin and is essentially a green summer squash that you're probably most used to seeing sliced and deep fried into zucchini "chips" or "poppers" that are laced with fat and calories. There's a lot more to the zucchini than a delivery mechanism for ranch dressing, though. Try some grilled in a sandwich or mixed into a stir-fry dish, and you'll see the true potential of this fruit—and gain all the health benefits in the process.

NUTRITIONAL INFORMATION

1 cup (120 g), chopped

Calories:	18
Fat:	0.16 g
Carbohydrate:	3.92 g
Dietary fiber:	1.8 g
Sugar:	0.45 g
Protein:	0.82 g

YOU NEED TO EAT THIS

WEIGHT LOSS

Low in calories and high in water content, zucchini will keep you away from snacking and will hydrate you at the same time. Because it is rich in fiber, it'll also keep you fuller longer while assisting in the weight-loss process.

BETTER SEX

Zucchinis are full of phytonutrients, which can reduce your symptoms of benign prostatic hypertrophy, which enlarges your prostate—ultimately resulting in difficult urination and poor sexual performance. Almost half the men with this condition report having a poor sex life, but diets rich in foods like zucchini helped them reclaim their function.

BETTER LOOKING SKIN

Zucchini's ability to increase manganese levels in your system spikes levels of an enzyme called superoxide dismutase, which has been proven to protect you from oxidative stress. It also helps produce proline, which triggers collagen formation resulting in better, healthier, and younger looking skin.

Easy Add-Ons to Your Diet

1. Slice zucchini and use as a dipper for salsa, guacamole, or other dip.
2. Slice lengthwise, drizzle with olive oil, and top with sea salt before grilling into a savory snack.
3. Include in egg scrambles.
4. With a spiralizer, make into zucchini noodles for an easy pasta swap.

★ = serving of green food

ZUCCHINI SMOOTHIE ★ ★

1 banana

1 large apple

1 zucchini

6 ounces (175 ml) coconut milk

Blend all of the ingredients on high, until smooth.

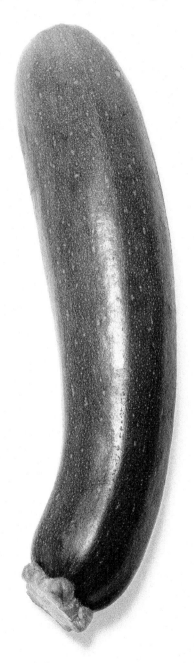

ZUCCHINI FRITTERS ★ ★

2 cups (240 g) shredded zucchini (about 2 medium zucchini)

3 eggs

1 tablespoon (7 g) coconut flour

½ teaspoon salt

¼ teaspoon pepper

Coconut oil

Shred the zucchini and ring dry with a paper towel. In a large bowl, beat the eggs together. Sift the coconut flour into the eggs and beat together. Mix the shredded zucchini, salt, and pepper together, and combine with the egg mixture. Pan fry in coconut oil.

SUPER-GREEN PESTO ★ ★ ★ ★

2 cups (80 g) basil

¼ cup (25 g) raw almonds

⅓ cup (80 ml) olive oil

4 cups (480 g) zucchini and spinach, finely chopped

Salt and pepper to taste

Place the basil and almonds into a blender or food processor. Pulse for 30 seconds. As blender is running, drizzle in olive oil through the top lid. Stop when the olive oil is gone and the pesto is completely mixed. Add salt and pepper to taste. Add the pesto to spaghetti squash or meat, such as steak or salmon. You can add 2 cloves of garlic or some lemon juice to jazz up the flavor of the pesto.

PREP TIP

• When preparing zucchini, make sure to remove both the top and bottom before cooking and wash thoroughly. Steaming lets your zucchini keep the most nutrients.

BUYING AND STORAGE TIPS

• Organic zucchini is your best bet to avoid genetically modified varieties that are laced with pesticides.

• Leave unwashed zucchini in an airtight container in your fridge for a week.

• If you want to freeze them, they'll keep longer, but they will get a little rubbery in the process.

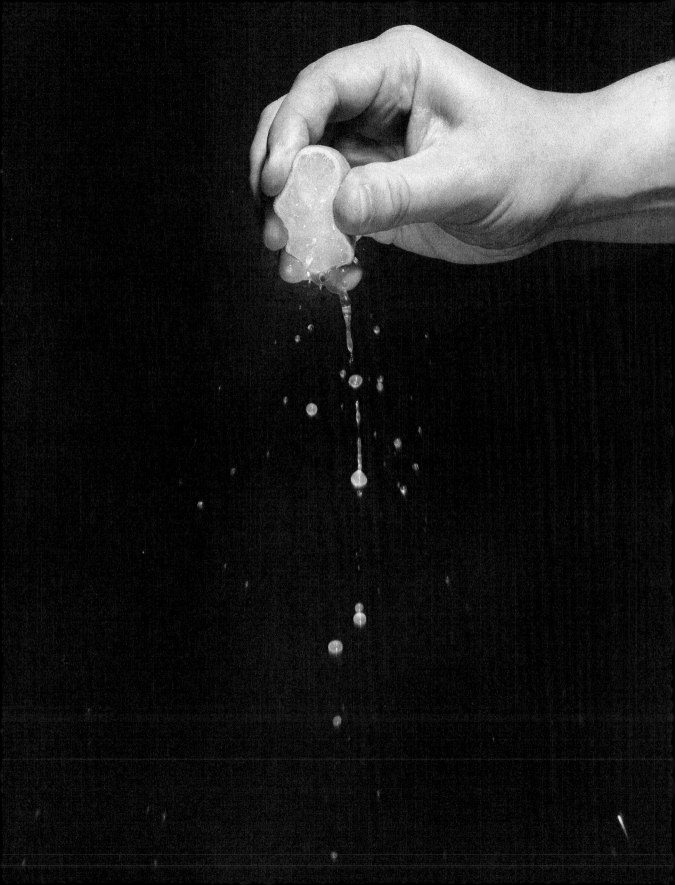

IT'S EASY BEING GREEN:
THE 3-DAY START UP

With this plan, you start slow by not changing anything in your diet. Instead, your mission is to simply add at least three green foods every day. Do this for three days to "try on" some green foods for size.

It's Easy Being Green is the best plan for you if you think it takes too many fork stabs to eat a salad, hate the taste of broccoli, or have not consumed anything green since 2003. This is the start of your green foods adventure.

"CHOOSE YOUR OWN ADVENTURE"

How you successfully complete this mission is up to you. On the next two pages, you'll find lists of numerous options for ways to add three or more green foods to your daily routine. For example, if you are an oatmeal-in-the-morning guy, you'll find suggestions for adding things like sliced pears or pumpkin seeds. Beyond breakfast, you'll find nutrient-packed green foods suggestions for everything from burger toppings to stir-fry add-ins.

YOUR MISSION
Add 3 green foods, 1 green snack, and 1 green smoothie for 3 days.

Oatmeal/Cereal

Kiwi, chopped or sliced
Pistachios
Pumpkin seeds
Pear, sliced
Green apples, chopped or sliced
Sautéed vegetables

Breakfast Sandwich

Green onions
Avocado
Pesto spread
Herbs

Scrambled Eggs/ Omelets

Spinach
Green onions
Kale
Avocado
Broccoli
Cilantro

Yogurt Parfait

Kiwi
Pistachios
Pumpkin seeds

Soup

Bok choy
Peas
Dill
Parsley
Broccoli sprouts

Salad

Beet greens
Grapes
Pistachios
Avocado
Pumpkin seeds
Turnip greens

Sandwich

Avocado
Romaine
Dill
Pesto spread
Broccoli sprouts
Blanched greens as wraps

Burrito Bowl/Tacos/ Fajitas/Quesadillas

Guacamole
Jalapeños
Cilantro
Green peppers
Tomatillos
Green onions

Egg/Tuna salad

Dill
Celery
Cucumber
Parsley
Pickles

Grilled Cheese

Spinach
Arugula
Avocado
Green onions
Parsley

Pasta
Zucchini noodles
Green beans
Green peas
Rosemary
Olive oil

Pizza
Oregano
Side salad on top
Green olives
Arugula
Spinach
Rosemary
Spinach, puréed and added
to sauce

Steak Sandwich
Jalapeños
Green peppers
Green onions

Steak and Potatoes
Brussels sprouts
Chives on baked potato

Chinese Food
Bok choy
Broccoli
Peas

Burger
Avocado slices
Romaine lettuce
Pickles
Rosemary mixed in ground beef
Chopped kale mixed in ground
beef

Chicken Stir Fry
Green peppers
Bok choy
Broccoli

Meatloaf/Meatballs
Thyme
Rosemary, mixed in ground beef
Kale, chopped and mixed in
ground beef
Green peas
Green peppers
Green onions

Mac and Cheese
Spinach, finely chopped
Broccoli

Salmon
Asparagus
Pesto
Zucchini
Leeks
Fennel
Broccoli

SAMPLE SNACK ADDS
Olives
Pumpkin seeds
Pistachios
Pickles
Green grapes
Green apple
Celery with almond butter
Broccoli with hummus
Green peppers strips
Cucumber slices
Honeydew melon
Kiwi
Pear slices

SAMPLE BEVERAGE ADDS
Cucumber water
Water with lime
Green tea
Green smoothie
Green juice

Still not getting it? (Don't worry, we won't tell anyone.) Well then, we've chosen your adventure for you: by pulling together some of our favorite recipe suggestions and turning them into a sample mission plan. You'll find recommendations for breakfast, lunch, and dinner, as well as snacks, smoothies, and more.

DAY ONE

EGGS AND STEAK WITH SAUTÉED SPINACH

BURRITO WITH GUACAMOLE

KALE BURGER AND FRIES

OLIVES

GREEN SMOOTHIE

GREEN TEA

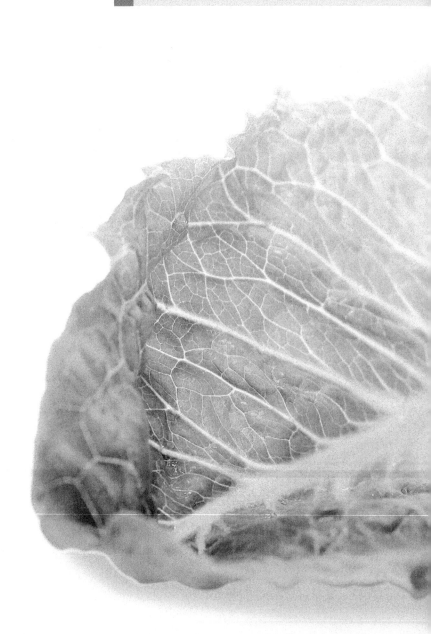

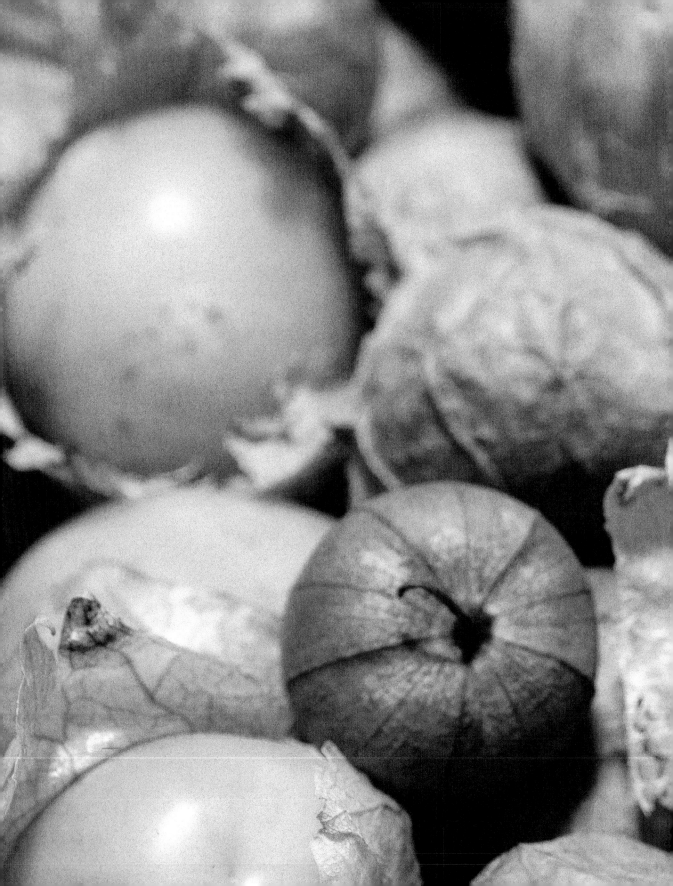

THE 7-DAY
QUICK-START CLEANSE

Let's get aggressive. You want quick gains, right? Follow this one-week intense plan to experience the benefits of green foods in all their glory. Your mission is to consume one green food serving for every 10 pounds (4.5 kg) your weight each day. The focus of this plan is on green foods that will enhance your body's natural detoxification mechanisms and give your digestion a chance to recover from the beat down you've been giving it for the last few months, or more. Hey guys, if your poop stinks, so does you diet. Time to giddy up.

If you're intrigued by the thought of a juice cleanse, but don't want to be hungry, this plan is for you.

Before any new diet plan you need to start by cleaning up house. Toxins can be a huge barrier to any health changes. With this cleanse, not only are you trying to eat foods that will literally bind to toxins, but also you want to support your body's natural detoxification pathways, so toxins can get the heck out.

Your main detoxification organs are your skin, kidneys, liver, and gall bladder. You excrete toxins through your urine and bowel movements, your skin, and even your hair! When any of these pathways are sluggish, toxins accumulate and create a whole host of problems such as low energy, weight gain, decreased sex drive, and more.

YOUR MISSION
Consume 1 green food serving for every 10 pounds (4.5 kg) of body weight per day for 1 week.

HOW IT WORKS

1. Consume 1 green food serving for every 10 pounds (4.5 kg) body weight for 7 days. This can be with meals, snacks, smoothies, or juices.
2. Eat as much of the approved foods as you'd like. There is no limit on quantity of approved food eaten during the 7 days.
3. Do not eat anything on the "Foods to Avoid" list (p. 147) for the entire duration of the plan.

Tip: Green smoothies and juices are the easiest ways to consume many green food servings in one sitting. We suggest adding a smoothie and a juice every day during the 7 days. For more advice on making smoothies and juices, see page 150.

WHY IT WORKS

Simply put, green foods are perfect for detoxification. They contain all the vitamins and minerals that are crucial to support your body's natural detoxification pathway. As a bonus, they work to heal your digestive tract and strengthen your immune system. The focus of this green food cleanse is to add these potent detoxifyers to your diet, especially cruciferous vegetables and herbs. But you'll also need to avoid the anti-green foods that are stressful on the body when consumed in excess (listed on p. 147). These foods, especially alcohol and refined sugar, may weaken your detoxification system, and wreak havoc on your digestion and immunity.

HERE'S WHY IT WORKS:

- Because there is no limit on the quantity of food, it includes an adequate amount of energy (calories) and nutrients to support the body's natural detoxification pathways. There is no starving needed.
- This is a plan that you could realistically continue to implement after the 7 days—for life. That is the true test of any diet or cleanse you try.
- The quality of the food is the main focus, with an emphasis on green foods that support detoxification, digestion, immunity, and energy. The more, the better!
- You take a break from foods that add or can potentially add a burden to the detoxification pathways in the short-term. Your body can use this time to heal and repair itself. Don't be afraid to delay reintroducing these "avoid" foods for as long as you can, and make sure they aren't consistently a part your diet going forward.

SEVEN SIGNS YOUR BODY COULD BENEFIT FROM A CLEANSE

- Fatigue, low energy
- Digestive issues (e.g., constipation, cramps, tired after meals)
- Migraines, headaches
- Low sex drive
- Anxiety, depression, mood swings
- Difficulty concentrating, brain fog
- Muscle or joint pain

Minimum Serving Sizes

Vegetables = ½ cup (50 g), cooked or raw
Leafy greens = 1 cup (100 g), raw
Fruit = ½ cup (50 g), raw or 1 medium piece
Nuts = 1 ounce (28 g) (size of your thumb)
Herbs = 1 tablespoon (15 g), fresh
Green tea = 8 ounces (235 ml)

When to Start a Cleanse

The best time to do a cleanse is when you don't have a lot of big social events or distractions that would tempt you into making poor food choices. You want to set yourself up for as much success as possible during the cleanse. Granted, there may never be a "perfect" time to start the cleanse, but think about when you can really ramp up your devotion to a wellness challenge like this and give it your best possible effort. Consider taking two to three days to prepare, plan meals, and shop for groceries, so you don't start off behind.

What You Need

This plan suggests one fresh juice and one smoothie every day. Because of this, you will need access to a juicer and a blender. If you don't have a juicer, you can buy juices at the store (look for the ones that are made fresh at the juice bar or Suja brand), plan to get them delivered (you'll want to make sure they're organic and unpasturized), or swap in an extra smoothie instead.

JUICERS WE LIKE
Breville
Hurom

BLENDERS WE LIKE
NutriBullet
Vitamix
Blendtec
Ninja

For more juicing tips, turn to page 150.

FOOD-BASED SUPPLEMENTS TO FACILITATE DETOXIFICATION

TAKE A MILK THISTLE supplement; this herb will help support the liver as it rids your body of toxins.

SUPPLEMENT WITH a green drink powder. This is not as good as fresh juices and smoothies, but an acceptable alternative when you don't have access to a blender.

IF YOU EXPERIENCE CONSTIPATION, try magnesium in powder or capsule form. Take before bed to promote bowel movements.

OTHER NATURAL DETOXIFICATION STRATEGIES

DRINK AT LEAST one-hundred ounces of water, ideally filtered water from a BPA-free container.

TRY AN INFRARED sauna treatment, although start slow if you have never used one before.

CHOOSE ORGANIC and GMO-free foods. Avoid eating out as much as possible.

REFRAIN FROM high-intensity training during the seven-day cleanse to focus on repair and detoxification.

SIP ON GREEN TEA with lemon and honey throughout the day. Drink hot or cold!

UP THE PARSLEY! This is an especially potent diuretic that will help excrete toxins as they are released and ready for exit.

AVOID EATING OUT as much as possible.

One week. That's all the time you need to commit to this adventure. Before you know it, you will be well on your way to a cleaner, healthier new you. Use this sample meal plan as your launching pad. Follow it exactly or customize it to your heart's desire. Take the lessons you learn during the week and apply them to the following week and beyond.

DAY ONE

APPLE CELERY JUICE ★ ★ ★   P.39

OATMEAL FOR MEN ★ ★   P.61

GREEN ON GREEN BISON BURGER ★ ★ ★ ★   P.91

ASIAN STIR FRY ★ ★ ★ ★   P.33

GREEN PEPPERS AND HUMMUS ★   P.61

DETOX SMOOTHIE ★ ★ ★   P.87

DAY FOUR

GREEN JUICE ★ ★ ★ ★   P.25

GREEN EGGS AND HAM ★ ★ ★ ★   P.35

PROTEIN AND SAUTÉED LEMON GARLIC COLLARD GREENS ★ ★   P.43

BEEF AND BROCCOLI STIR FRY ★ ★ ★ ★   P.35

STUFFED OLIVES ★   P.143

KALE AND GREEN APPLE SMOOTHIE ★ ★ ★   P.71

DAY SEVEN

PHYLL UP JUICE ★ ★ ★ ★ ★ ★   P.87

WAFFLE BREAKFAST SANDWICH ★   P.27

CHICKEN AND SPICY GREEN BEANS ★ ★ ★   P.53

BAKED GREEN PEPPERS ★   P.61

AVOCADO PUDDING ★ ★ ★   P.27

TROPICAL SMOOTHIE ★ ★ ★   P.25

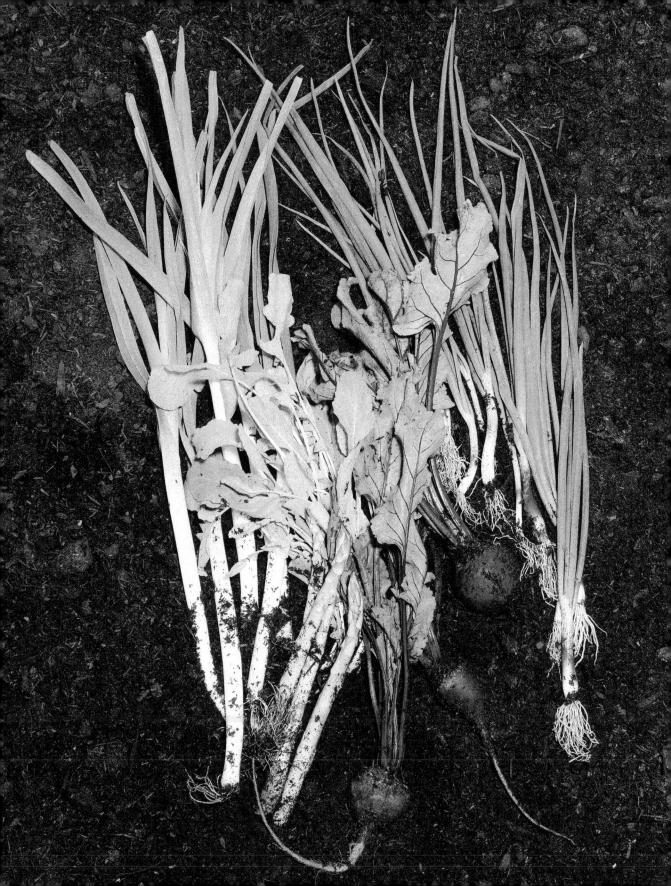

THE 30-DAY
GREEN FOODS DIET CHALLENGE:
GREENS FOR GAINS

This 30-day plan is a healthy, clean eating plan, where you have to keep the amount of green foods you eat at a minimum of ten servings per day. We hope that this challenge can be something you can keep up past day thirty. Along with the increase in greenness, you'll see gains in flavor, gains in culinary confidence, and of course, all those other amazing gains that come with eating more of nature's best.
Think better energy, more productivity, improved sex drive, immunity made of steel, and a complete and total domination of life.

YOUR MISSION
Eat a minimum of
10 servings a day for a
month—and beyond

We'll highlight specific recipes found in this book you can add for specific gains you are looking for, and you will also get a sample fifteen-day plan you can double up on, or just use as a sample to make your own thirty-day challenge.

We'll suggest numerous recipes found throughout the profiles of the 50 Green Superfoods that will provide you with inspiration and motivation for your 30-day mission. The recipes are divided into handy categories, such as Smoothies, Juices, Breakfasts, Entrees, Sides and Dressings, Salads, Beverages, and Snacks. You will also find a sample 15-day plan followed by a blank meal planner template you can use to customize and design the second half of the challenge.

We also suggest you flip ahead to the Resources section, beginning on page 143. There you'll find a guide listing the top foods for achieving a half dozen very specific goals. Whether you're looking for the green foods most likely to improve your sexual performance or decrease stress, you'll have them all indexed in easy-to-use lists. You'll also find lists of other foods to enjoy--and foods to avoid--as well as a treasure trove of tips for everything from eating out and eating clean to juicing, making smoothies, and more.

The Greens for Gains plan is an extremely flexible plan, focusing on adding nutrient-dense real foods to your diet. with an emphasis on the green superfoods featured in this book. Clinical research and scientific studies back up the true power of green foods and the positive impact they have on your health and wellness.

WHY IT WORKS

SUPPORTS YOUR HEALTH

The plan was designed to support male health from the inside out. You'll improve your prostate health and boost your prevention of prostate cancer. You'll handle chronic or low-grade inflammation, the precursor of many chronic diseases, with anti-inflammatory herbs and healthy fats. You will improve your body composition by decreasing dietary stressors, a common obstacle to fat loss. You will gain energy, mental clarity, and more to have you feeling younger than you have ever felt.

KEEPS THINGS SIMPLE

We keep this plan straight to the point with simple ingredients and easy-to-follow directions. Every recipe features at least one green food and is four ingredients or less, excluding cooking oil and simple seasoning. The directions are short, but the result will make you feel like a culinary genius.

TASTES GREAT

Why eat food that you don't enjoy? With these recipes, there's no need for chemical flavor enhancers! Simple seasoning and high-quality real food heighten the flavor of every recipe. Herbs and spices add a punch of nutrients along with tastebud-pleasing taste.

DISCLAIMERS

Serving Sizes: This meal plan is not one-size-fits-all. Rather, it is a template and starting point. Serving sizes are general recommendations and will vary based on your weight, activity level, and goals.

Variety: You want some degree of variety in your diet to ensure you are getting a well-rounded amount of nutrients. However, there is no shame in rotating your top three to five meals, snacks, smoothies, and juices. Routine is never a bad thing as long as the routine is good.

Hydration: Because green foods are fiber powerhouses, as your green food intake goes up, your water intake must also go up. Consider adding a pinch of unrefined sea salt, lime, cucumber, or mint to your water as well.

Additional Resources: Be sure to reference the Resources section (p. 143) for additional ideas and strategies to follow the Greens for Gains plan.

Tip: Green smoothies and juices are the easiest ways to consume many green food servings in one sitting. We suggest adding a smoothie and a juice every day during the 7 days. For more, refer to the "Smoothie Tips" and "Basic Smoothie Builder" sections, on page 150.

ENTRÉES

DILL SALMON BURGERS ★   P.47

BAKED GREEN PEPPERS ★   P.61

PISTACHIO-CRUSTED SALMON ★ ★   P.93

ASIAN STIR FRY ★ ★ ★   P.33

BEEF AND BROCCOLI STIR FRY ★ ★ ★ ★   P.35

BASIL ARTICHOKE MEATBALLS ★ ★ ★   P.21

PUMPKIN SEED CRUSTED CHICKEN ★ ★   P.95

CHICKEN AND CHARD BOWL ★ ★   P.111

BRAISED SAUERKRAUT WITH BRATWURST ★   P.103

LEMON THYME FISH HOT POCKET ★ ★ ★   P.113

STRAWBERRY BASIL CHICKEN ★ ★   P.29

GRASS-FED STEAK FAJITAS   P.61

SLOW COOKER CHICKEN TACOS ★   P.69

GREEN ON GREEN BISON BURGER ★ ★ ★ ★   P.91

ON-THE-GO LUNCH ★ ★   P.93

SIDES

DIJON TURNIP GREENS ★ ★   P.117

LEMON THYME MUSHROOMS ★   P.113

GRILLED ROMAINE AND PROSCIUTTO ★ ★   P.97

SAUTÉED LEEKS ★   P.75

BACON BALSAMIC BRUSSELS SPROUTS ★ ★ ★ ★   P.37

HOMEMADE SAUERKRAUT ★   P.103

SAUTÉED CELERY ★ ★ ★ ★ ★   P.39

CILANTRO CAULIFLOWER RICE ★ ★   P.41

SAUTÉED LEMON GARLIC COLLARD GREENS ★ ★   P.43

HONEY CASHEW GREEN BEANS ★ ★   P.53

GREEN BEAN FRIES ★ ★   P.53

SPICY GREEN BEANS ★ ★ ★   P.53

GARLIC DIJON ARTICHOKES ★ ★   P.21

BALSAMIC CHARD ★ ★   P.111

DULSE MISO SOUP ★ ★   P.105

PROSCIUTTO-WRAPPED ASPARAGUS ★ ★   P.25

SAUER-SLAW ★   P.103

BASIL-INFUSED BRUSCHETTA ★ ★   P.29

SAUTÉED GRAPES AND GOAT CHEESE ★ ★ ★   P.55

AVOCADO-CILANTRO RICE ★ ★ ★   P.41

PAN-FRIED ASPARAGUS ★   P.25

ENERGY-PACKED GREENS ★ ★ ★   P.43

SAUCES AND DRESSINGS

LEMON MINT DRESSING ★ ★ ★   P.79

OLIVE OIL VINAIGRETTE ★   P.81

FIVE-MINUTE ITALIAN DRESSING ★ ★ ★   P.85

LEMON PARSLEY SAUCE ★ ★   P.87

TOMATILLO SALSA VERDE ★ ★ ★   P.115

ARUGULA PESTO ★ ★   P.23

AVOCADO VINAIGRETTE ★ ★ ★ ★   P.27

BASIL AVOCADO SAUCE ★ ★ ★ ★   P.29

BASIL VINAIGRETTE ★ ★   P.29

CREAMY CILANTRO SAUCE ★ ★ ★ ★   P.40

AVOCADO SPAGHETTI SAUCE ★ ★ ★   P.27

SUPER-GREEN PESTO ★ ★ ★   P.119

SALADS

SEAWEED SALAD ★ ★   P.105

OREGANO WHITE BEAN SALAD ★ ★   P.85

MINT MELON SALAD ★ ★ ★   P.67

KIWI LEEK APPLE SALAD ★ ★ ★   P.75

PEAR AND WALNUT SALAD ★ ★   P.89

ROSEMARY GREEN PEA SALAD ★ ★ ★ ★   P.59

BRUSSELS SPROUTS SALAD ★ ★ ★ ★ ★ ★   P.37

CELERY SLAW ★ ★ ★ ★ ★ ★ ★   P.39

PROTEIN SALAD ★ ★ ★ ★ ★ ★   P.39

AVOCADO CHICKEN SALAD ★ ★ ★ ★   P.27

WATERMELON AND BASIL SALAD ★ ★ ★ ★   P.29

SUPER-GREEN SALAD ★ ★ ★ ★ ★   P.77

ARUGULA SALAD ★ ★ ★   P.23

KALE SUPER SALAD ★ ★ ★   P.81

BEVERAGES

THYME TEA ★   P.113

PRODUCTIVI-TEA ★ ★   P.63

FENNEL MINT TEA ★ ★   P.49

LIME AND MINT WATER ★ ★   P.79

MINT TEA ★   P.79

GREEN TEA ★   P.63

CUCUMBER WATER ★   P.45

SNACKS

CHILI LIME PUMPKIN SEEDS ★ ★   P.77

ZUCCHINI FRITTERS ★ ★   P.119

OVERNIGHT REFRIGERATOR PICKLES ★ ★   P.91

BOURBON MAPLE PISTACHIOS ★   P.93

OLIVE SALSA ★ ★   P.83

OLIVE TAPENADE ★ ★   P.83

GREEN APPLE SALSA ★ ★ ★ ★   P.55

AVOCADO PUDDING ★ ★ ★   P.27

KALE CHIPS ★ ★   P.71

DILL VEGETABLE DIP ★   P.47

GUACAMOLE ★ ★   P.27

STUFFED COLLARD GREENS ★ ★ ★ ★   P.43

ARUGULA-STUFFED TURKEY ROLL UPS ★   P.23

GREEN APPLE AND CELERY AND ALMOND BUTTER ★ ★   P.23

PISTACHIOS AND GRAPES ★ ★   P.55

GREEN TRAIL MIX ★ ★   P.55

STUFFED OLIVES ★   P.83

CHIA PUDDING WITH PISTACHIOS ★   P.93

MINI PICKLE SANDWICHES ★   P.91

SARDINES ★   P.81

DAY 1-15

This challenge is set up as a way to ensure you get ten servings of greens everyday. We've outlined fifteen days in this sample meal plan so you can see how best to balance your meal choices. You can choose to follow this plan once and make up your own for the second half of the challenge, follow this plan twice to fill out your thirty days, or make up your own mind for every meal — making sure you reach your ten green foods per day quota.

DAY ONE

EGG BANCAKES WITH PURÉED KIWI ★ ★   P.73

PEAR AND WALNUT SALAD ★ ★ **WITH SLICED GRILLED CHICKEN**   P.89

BAKED GREEN PEPPERS ★   P.61

SPINBERRY SMOOTHIE ★ ★ ★   P.107

MINI PICKLE SANDWICHES ★   P.91

GREEN TEA ★   P.63

DAY FOUR

GREEN EGGS ★   P.71 **WITH SIDE OF GREEN GRAPES** ★   P.55

ROSEMARY GREEN PEA SALAD ★ ★ ★ ★ **WITH SLICED GRILLED PORK LOIN**   P.59

GRILLED TILAPIA WITH GRILLED ROMAINE AND PROSCIUTTO ★ ★   P.97

PISTACHIOS AND GRAPES ★   P.55

MINT TEA ★   P.79

DAY SEVEN

WAFFLE BREAKFAST SANDWICH ★   P.27

SAUTÉED LEEKS ★ **WITH GRILLED GRASS-FED NY STRIP STEAK**   P.75

BEEF AND BROCCOLI STIR FRY ★ ★ ★ ★   P.35

ROMAINE AND CARROT JUICE ★ ★   P.97

PLANTAIN CHIPS AND GUACAMOLE ★ ★   P.27

DAY TEN

CHIA PUDDING WITH PISTACHIOS ★   P.93

BBQ PULLED PORK WITH AVOCADO RICE ★ ★ ★   P.41

GRILLED STEAK WITH BACON BALSAMIC BRUSSELS SPROUTS ★ ★ ★ ★   P.37

KALE CHIPS ★ ★   P.71

DAY THIRTEEN

EGG STUFFED GREEN PEPPERS ★   P.61

AVOCADO CHICKEN SALAD ★ ★ ★ ★   P.27

PUMPKIN SEED CRUSTED CHICKEN ★ ★   P.95

CARROT ASPARAGUS TOMATO JUICE ★ ★   P.25

GREEN APPLE AND CELERY WITH ALMOND BUTTER ★ ★   P.143

DAY 16-30

Repeat the Day 1–15 meal plan or create your own plan to eat ten green food servings per day. Use these pages to keep track of your green food intakes.

DAY SIXTEEN

DAY NINETEEN

DAY TWENTY-TWO

DAY TWENTY-FIVE

DAY TWENTY-EIGHT

DAY SEVENTEEN

DAY TWENTY

DAY TWENTY-THREE

DAY TWENTY-SIX

DAY TWENTY-NINE

DAY EIGHTEEN

DAY TWENTY-ONE

DAY TWENTY-FOUR

DAY TWENTY-SEVEN

DAY THIRTY

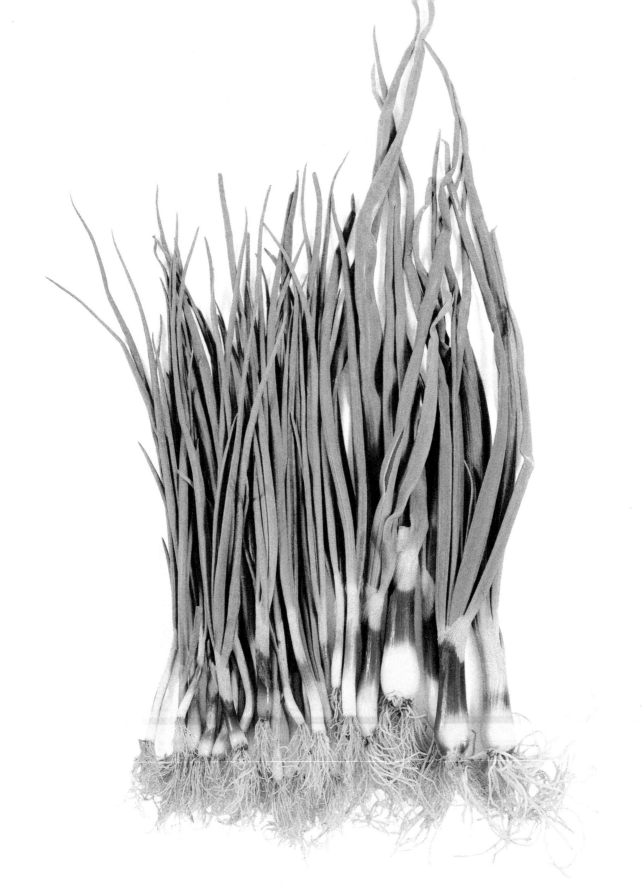

RESOURCES

Improve Your Athletic Performance

Eating green could be the difference between completing a workout and crushing it.

Muscle and athletic performance come down to optimizing your hormonal balance and recovering properly from strenuous training.

Jalapeños
Kiwi
Limes
Spirulina
Spinach

Rev-Up Sexual Performance

Eat like your manhood depends on it. Because it does!

Healthy sources of fat provide raw material for your male hormones, and other highlighted green foods are a good source of nitric oxide, which improves blood flow (to you know where).

Olives
Olive oil
Pistachios
Pumpkin seeds
Avocado
Zucchini
Collard greens
Spinach
Celery
Green onions

Healthy Hair

Healthy hair growth on the outside starts on the inside. Consume green foods that support digestion so you can benefit from their key healthy hair nutrients.

Sauerkraut
Pickles
Mint
Arugula
Cucumber
Beet greens
Fennel
Oregano
Artichokes
Basil

Perk-Up and Be Productive

Enjoy these surprising sources of sustained energy.

Green peppers
Green tea
Seaweed
Avocado

Go Stress Free

Fight the war against physical and mental stress.

Green apples
Spinach
Green peas
Turnip greens
Leeks
Rosemary

Detox Like a Champ

Get a daily dose of these go-to greens for keeping it clean.

Brussels sprouts
Bok choy
Kale
Parsley
Asparagus
Broccoli
Cilantro

Organic Vegetables

Assist your liver, your #1 detox organ, in its natural detoxification mechanisms.

Artichokes
Arugula
Asparagus
Bamboo shoots
Bean sprouts
Beets
Beet greens
Bell peppers (red, yellow, green)
Broad beans
Broccoli
Brussels sprouts
Cabbage
Carrots
Cassava
Cauliflower
Celery
Chives

Cilantro
Collard greens
Cucumber
Dandelion greens
Eggplant
Endive
Fennel
Garlic
Ginger (fresh)
Green beans
Jalapeño peppers
Jicama
Kale
Kohlrabi
Leeks
Mushrooms
Mustard greens
Okra

Onions (green, white, purple)
Parsley
Radicchio
Radishes
Shallots
Spaghetti squash
Spinach
Sugar snap peas
Summer squash (yellow, zucchini)
Sweet potatoes
Swiss chard
Tomatoes
Turnip greens
Turnips
Watercress
Winter squash (acorn, butternut, pumpkin)

Organic Fruits

Clean up cell damage and boost antioxidant intake.

Apples
Apricots (fresh)
Avocados
Bananas
Blackberries
Blueberries
Boysenberries
Cherries
Elderberries
Gooseberries
Grapefruit

Grapes
Kiwi fruit
Lemons
Limes
Loganberries
Mangos
Melons
Nectarines
Oranges
Papayas
Peaches

Pears
Pineapple
Plums
Pomegranates
Prunes (dried plums)
Raspberries
Strawberries
Tangerines
Watermelon

NOTE: The 50 Green Superfoods profiled in this book appear in **bold**.

Pastured Meat and Poultry

Detoxify with essential amino acids from clean protein sources.

Beef, pasture-raised,
100 percent grass-fed
Bison, 100 percent grass-fed
Chicken, pasture-raised
Duck, free-range
Turkey, free-range

Deli meats, nitrite-free, organic
Eggs (whole, organic,
pastured)
Lamb, pasture-raised
Goat, pasture-raised
Pork, pasture-raised

Wild game (venison, elk)
Bacon, pasture-raised,
uncured, additive-free
Ghee, clarified butter

Dairy

Ghee
Clarified butter

Other dairy products, grass-fed,
full-fat and , ideally, low
temperature pasturized

Sustainable Seafood

Improve mental health and focus while detoxifying.

Albacore Tuna (troll- or pole-
caught, from the U.S. or
British Columbia)
Freshwater Coho Salmon
(farmed in tank systems,
from the U.S.)

Oysters (farmed)
Pacific Sardines
(wild-caught)
Rainbow Trout (farmed)

Salmon (wild-caught,
from Alaska)
Shrimp, wild (from Maine)

Organic Nuts, Seeds, & Oils

Achieve hormonal balance and support cellular repair,
while keeping your immune system in check.

Coconut oil (refined for neutral;
unrefined for flavor)
Brazil nuts
Coconut milk
Cod liver oil (ideally fermented)
**Extra-virgin olive oil
(unheated)**

Fresh coconut
Grapeseed oil
Ground flaxseeds
Macadamia nuts
Nut butters
Olives
Safflower mayonnaise

Sesame oil
Sprouted nuts (almonds,
cashews, walnuts, pecans)
Sprouted seeds (pumpkin,
sunflower, sesame)
Unrefined flaxseed oil
Unrefined sesame oil

Fermented Foods

Strengthen your digestion to improve nutrient absorption, energy, and immunity.

Kombucha
Pickles
Sauerkraut
Fermented salsa

Kim Chi
Apple cider vinegar
Cultured vegetables
Coconut water kefir

Fermented ketchup
Fermented mustard
Wine, organic, no sulfites added

Herbs & Condiments

These superfoods pack a whole lot of power in just a little pinch.

Parsley
Cilantro
Ginger
Garlic

Thyme
Oregano
Mint
Rosemary

Sage
Chamomile
Cayenne pepper

Superfoods

Fight inflammation and improve health from the inside out with small, but mighty superfoods.

Green tea
Raw apple cider vinegar
Unrefined sea salt
Unfiltered raw, local honey

Organic Grade B maple syrup
Homemade bone broth
Dark chocolate (70% or more
   cocoa or cacao)

Seaweed (dulse, kelp)
Spirulina

Legumes

Black beans
Chickpeas
French beans (flageolets)
Great Northern beans
Green peas
Kidney beans
Lentils
Lima beans
Navy and Pinto beans
Split peas
White beans
Yellow beans
Yams

Grains

Brown rice
Buckwheat groats (kasha)
Bulgur (tabouli)
Gluten-free oats
Quinoa (a grain-like seed)
White rice
Wild rice

FOODS TO AVOID

MAN-MADE CHEMICALS MSG, high fructose corn syrup, food dyes, artificial sweeteners, synthetic vitamins, minerals and supplements; or industrialized oils (e.g., soybean oil, corn oil, canola oil)

PROCESSED GLUTEN AND GRAINS Store-bought bread, crackers, anything with "enriched flour"

REFINED SUGARS Table sugar, evaporated cane sugar, filtered honey, agave syrup

FACTORY FARMED ANIMALS AND SEAFOOD Conventionally raised beef and chicken, given antibiotics and hormones, most farmed fish; conventional dairy products from factory-farmed cows.

LOW-FAT FOODS Low-fat yogurts, low-fat milk, margarine spreads

ALCOHOL

Optional Foods to Avoid

CAFFEINE (or significantly reduce, and only use organic)

GRAINS (rice, quinoa; choose sweet potatoes or potatoes instead)

LEGUMES (beans, hummus) Note any digestive stress and avoid, if necessary.

RED MEAT (While red meat is not necessarily on the "do-not-eat" list, it is an option to take a seven-day hiatus and give your liver a temporary break.)

1. Your success starts before the meal. Don't arrive famished and unprepared.

- Eat two to three hours before your dining experience so that you don't arrive famished with a low blood sugar, and give in to quick treats.
- As always, eat balanced throughout the day rather than "saving calories" for what you think will be a big meal at the end of your day.
- Research the menu beforehand so you can have time to review the menu and order with confidence.
- Many restaurants will post gluten-free menus online, but not in the restaurant.
- Tell your waiter at the beginning of the meal that you will not be ordering dessert, so that you aren't tempted at the end of the meal.

2. No matter what, get in the greens!

- Double up on steamed or raw vegetables (preferably without any processed sauces)! Skip the starchy or processed gluten-containing sides.
- Other menu items may have vegetable sides that you would enjoy. Ask the waiter to mix and match sides in a create-your-own entrée. Then pair with a clean protein and a healthy fat!
- Order a salad. ALWAYS. Choose balsamic vinegar and/or oil. There is almost always added sugar in the ranch, Italian, or house dressings.
- For optimal digestion of meat, it is best to consume your salad or vegetables with or after consuming the meat.

3. Ask and you shall receive. Be creative in your orders.

- Ask for sandwiches with a lettuce wrap instead.
- There's always steak, chicken, or other meats on the menu! Keep it simple. Poultry or lean beef is better if the beef is organic, pastured, and 100 percent grass-fed.
- Ask the waiter to put all sauces on the side, as they have many sources of hidden sugar.
- In pasta dishes, ask for the pasta fixings to be served on a plate of sautéed or fresh spinach instead of noodles.
- Mix a healthier side dish from one meal with the main course from another.
- Request bottles of olive oil and vinegar to use as salad or vegetable dressing.
- Ask about hidden ingredients that may not be on the menu. Double check your choices with the waiter to make sure there are no other ingredients than what is described.

4. When you can't control the quality, control the quantity.

- It's all about portion control when eating out. Not only are portions too large for one meal, but they are also not high quality. When you can't control the quality, control the quantity.
- Eat protein the size of your smartphone, carbohydrates the size of your fist, and fill the other half of your plate with salad and vegetables.
- If portions are too large, ask the waiter to split the portion in half before it arrives at the table.
- Order an appetizer and small salad instead of a main course to better control the amount of food placed in front of you.

5. Avoid the "free" foods.

Free fillers like the bread basket, after-dinner candy, or free refills are mindless ways to eat food you didn't mean to consume. Save your appetite (and spare your blood sugar) by skipping the freebies.

6. Choose the best of the worst.

Steer clear of anything with the words fried, creamy, crispy, or battered.

7. Be mindful and mind your own business.

- Eat slowly. Chew your food completely and savor the flavor.
- Give yourself visual cues to remind you that you are done. Put your napkin and utensils over your plate to let your mind know that you are done.
- Don't let the food linger. Ask the waiter to take your plate as soon as you are satisfied.
- One easy tip is to chew a piece of gum after you are done eating to avoid mindless nibbling at your leftovers.
- Dining out should still be a fun experience, but choose your top one indulgence (e.g., bread, a cocktail, or your favorite dessert, not all three).
- Choose your splurge and really savor it. It should be something you really love, not just like. Enjoy the flavor to the fullest and have zero guilt!
- Keep your eyes on your own plate and don't fret about what everyone else is ordering or what people think of your order. You create your own dining experience with your own intentions. Don't let their choices mess you up!

Bonus Tips on Alcohol

- Red wine is always a great option. It's rich in antioxidants and can support cardiovascular health due to its resveratrol content.
- Mix in a water! Drink an alcoholic drink followed by a glass of water. Finish the water before you order your next drink. This will improve your alcohol metabolism and prevent you from getting too buzzed.
- Water with lemon or lime is better than just water. This helps to alkalize the blood and balance the acidic effects of alcohol.
- Try sticking to a two drink maximum per night.

SMOOTHIE TIPS

- Smoothies are blended whole foods (using a blender).
- Add lemon to a smoothie to prevent oxidation so you can save a serving for later.
- If your blender is not that powerful, remove the stems from your greens, like kale and swiss chard.
- Blend in stages, blending greens and liquid first, then adding the rest.
- Purée long enough for everything to be completely incorporated.
- Basic smoothie = 2 cups (200 g) greens + 2 cups (475 ml) liquid base + 2 cups (200 g) frozen or fresh fruit.
- It can be tempting to go light on the greens and heavy on the fruit. You know you are making the smoothie correctly, and including enough greens, when the smoothie is actually bright green in color.

BASIC SMOOTHIE BUILDER

BASE: water, coconut water, green tea, coconut, or almond milk

GREENS: spinach, kale, collards, beet greens, swiss chard

FRUIT: berries, avocado, kiwi, green apple, pear, honeydew melon

BOOST: spirulina, dulse flakes, nut butters, cinnamon, raw cacao

SWEETENER: honey, chopped dates, maple syrup

JUICING TIPS

- Juices are extracted liquid from whole foods (using a juicer).
- Juices are best consumed first thing in the morning on an empty stomach.
- Add lemon to juice to prevent oxidation so you can save a serving for later.
- When storing the juice, fill up to the top of the container and use a tight lid, to slow down oxidation.
- Use organic, especially for juicing.
- Wait at least two hours after a meal to drink a green juice, and wait twenty minutes after drinking a green juice to consume a meal
- Ideally, consume the juice as soon as you can after making it.
- If you decide to store your juice, remember to keep it refrigerated at all times before consuming.
- Juice isn't a meal replacement and should be consumed like a supplement within twenty minutes before a complete meal.
- Different types of juicers produce varying amounts of juice from your ingredients. The recipes here are estimates of how much whole produce it would take to produce a single serving of the recipe.

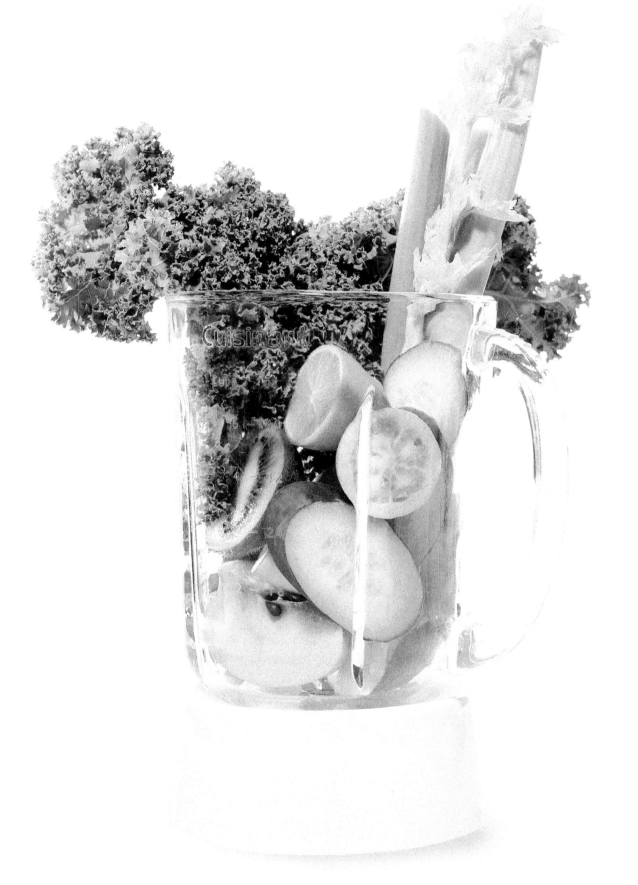

DIRTY DOZEN

Thanks to pesticides, some foods just aren't as healthy. The list below are the worst culprits. Choose organic for any fruit or vegetable on the Dirty Dozen list.

Apples
Celery
Red bell peppers
Peaches
Strawberries
Nectarines (imported)
Grapes
Spinach
Lettuce
Cucumber
Blueberries (domestic)
Potatoes

The following may contain pesticide residues of special concern:

Green beans
Kale/Greens

Source: Environmental Working Group

CLEAN FIFTEEN

The Clean Fifteen lists the least sprayed conventional produce that is acceptable to consume non-organic, although organic is still recommended.

Sweet Corn
Onions
Pineapple
Avocado
Cabbage
Sweet Peas- frozen
Papaya
Mangos
Asparagus
Eggplant
Kiwi
Grapefruit
Cantaloupe
Sweet Potato
Mushrooms

ACKNOWLEDGMENTS

This book would not have happened without the support of my family. Any strength or talent I may have is borne from them and made better through their support. I would also like to thank all the friends and colleagues who helped along the way: James, Tom, Dean, Jessica, John, Lisa, Rico, Derek and Charlie. Also, special thanks to my co-author Jenny Westerkamp who made this book more informative and more fun with each passing day. And, ultimately, thanks to you, the reader, for picking this up and letting the words, pictures, and ideas herein impact your quest for better health. Also, I thank God for letting me put words on paper and allowing me to live my dream. -MDM

Thank you to my mom, dad, brothers—Tim, Pat, Jim, Matt, and Jack—and sister-in-law, Kate, for their never-ending love and support. They always answer my questions, book-related or otherwise, with the blunt honesty that I need. I thank God for them, and for all the countless blessings in my life. I also want to express immense gratitude for my co-author Michael De Medeiros. His guidance and expertise were indispensable throughout this entire process. Finally, thank you to my focus-group participants, composed of male friends, cousins, uncles, former classmates, and Twitter followers. They tested many variations of nutrition plans and recipes, and provided valuable feedback and insights. -JW

We could not have completed this book without the hard work and dedication of our intern team: Katie Abrahamson, Yuhin Auyeung, Kelly Cassidy, Molika Chea, Morgan Clift, Lauren Gerker, Alison Hadavi, Stephanie Johnson, Adrienne Kahn, Christine Lally, Emily O'Neil, Anna Pleet, Suzy Podleyon, and Taylor Wessel.

We would also like to thank our photographer Robert Reiff and Chef Sandra Cordero for their aid in making this book look as amazing as it does. In addition, a huge thanks goes to all the unsung heroes at our publisher who worked tirelessly to make this book happen. Thanks all!

ABOUT THE AUTHORS

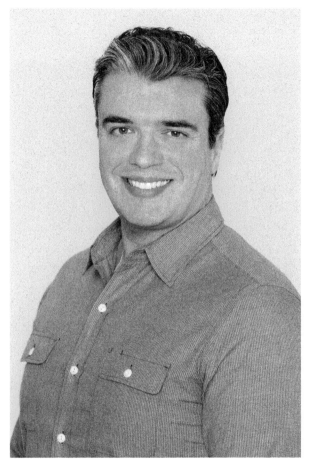

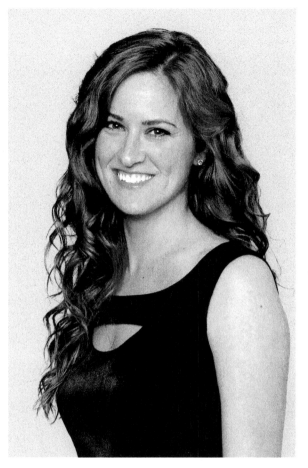

MICHAEL DE MEDEIROS is the former vice president and editor in chief of *Men's Fitness magazine*, former editor in chief of *Maximum Fitness* magazine, and author of thirteen books, including historical biographies, educational textbooks, and active health and fitness books. He has been nominated and shortlisted for several awards, including best book and best book in a series for Weigl publishers.

JENNY WESTERKAMP, R.D., is a holistic-minded registered dietitian, speaker, and author. She is the nutritionist for Kitchfix and an advisor for On Demand Dietitian. Previously, she worked with professional and collegiate athletes across the country and was president of Chicago Food and Nutrition Network. She has been interviewed for national media outlets and has spoken to groups on wellness, men's health, sports nutrition, and social media.

INDEX

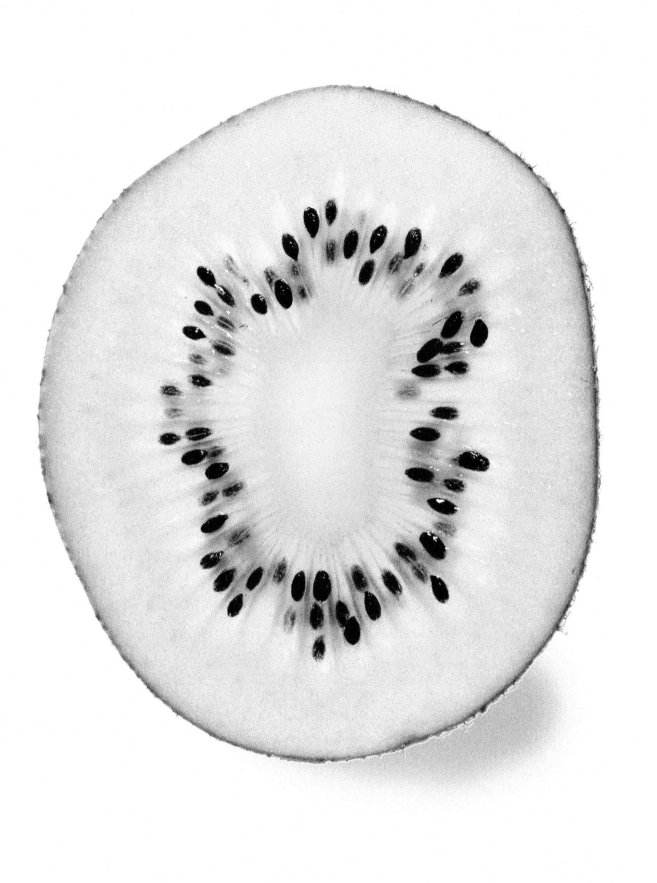

Don't miss these other Fair Winds Press books!

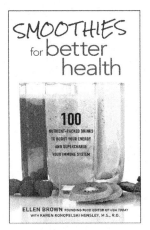

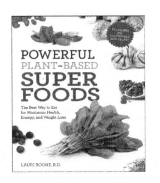

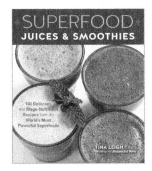

Smoothies for Better Health
Ellen Brown and Karen Konopelski Hensley
ISBN: 978-1-59233-542-8

Powerful Plant-Based Superfoods
Lauri Boone
ISBN: 978-1-59233-534-3

Superfood Juices and Smoothies
Tina Leigh
ISBN: 978-1-59233-604-3

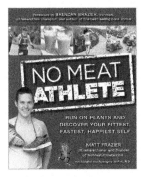

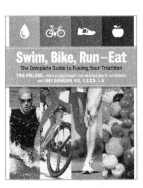

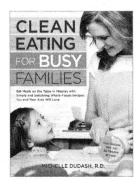

No Meat Athlete
Matt Frazier and Matt Ruscigno
ISBN: 978-1-59233-578-7

Swim, Bike, Run—Eat
Tom Holland and Amy Goodson
ISBN: 978-1-59233-606-7

Clean Eating for Busy Families
Michelle Dudash
ISBN: 978-1-59233-514-5

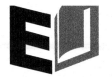

Our books are available as E-Books, too!
Many of our bestselling titles are now available as E-Books.
Visit www.Qbookshop.com to find links to e-vendors!

CPSIA information can be obtained
at www.ICGtesting.com
Printed in the USA
LVOW05s1238171016
PP11485700001B/5/P